Healthy Happy You

By

Balraj Aggarwal

Dedication

This book is dedicated to four very special persons in my life who have provided me with an incredible spark. My father taught me many Yoga and meditation exercises. My son, Rajat Kumar, guided me through the intricacies of the exercises and poses in a health club setting. My daughter, Tuhina A. Ruff, helped me accomplish my dream of writing this book with her love, sacrifices, and positive outlook. My wife, Meena, has always shown me the light and direction. They all are my real joy and I am blessed to have them in my life.

Love   Live   Laugh

Disclaimer

The material in this book is intended to unfold some guidelines for positive thinking that lead to achieving happiness, staying healthy and alert, reducing stress, and establishing and following a safe and effective exercise program. However, the reader is advised to consult his or her physician before beginning any exercise program. This is especially true for a reader with pre-existing medical problem(s).

Many professionals in the fields of positive thinking and physical fitness may have differing opinions; the author is providing information that is based on his own experiences and those of his family, friends, and individuals in or outside the classes taken on these subjects.

The author, publisher, and editors cannot be held responsible if the guidelines provided in this book do not work for you for any other reason including error, omission, dated material, or adverse outcomes that might result by following the information and exercises provided.

The exercise program(s) in this book are for self-care, however, you may prefer to practice them under the supervision and guidance of a licensed practitioner.

WARNING: You are strongly advised to always play it safe. If at any time you feel light-headed, unstable, dizzy, or sick, STOP the exercise to recover and stabilize yourself.

My primary personal objective is to help you. This book is intended to have a broad approach and be used by you and others. The activities are

Love   Live   Laugh

simple to practice and are meant to help middle-aged people and senior citizens reduce stress and live a stress-free, healthy and happy life.

Information in this book is not intended to replace the advice of your physician, dietician, or a physical therapist. *Healthy Happy You* is meant to provide you with the knowledge you need to make sound decisions. The author disclaims any liability for the decisions you may make based on the information in this book.

I am neither a physician, dietician, nor a physical therapist. I am a scientist, an analyst, and a logician who explores and synthesizes the causes practically that may be applicable to your physical and/or psychological reasoning or implications. I want to find solutions to help you reduce medications, and whenever possible I apply the solutions to myself before suggesting them to anyone else. Again, the coverage in this book is based upon my own experiences and knowledge.

Essence

The core essence of this book emanates from

a Sanskrit Sloka (verse) of Vedas:

"SHARIR MADYAM KHALU DHARMA SADHANAM"

This Sloka means:

It is our sacred duty to protect our body's health.
Keep mind and body in top shape.

As Jim Rohn, America's foremost business philosopher puts it:

Treat your body like a temple, not a woodshed. The mind and body work together. Your body needs to be a good support system for the mind and the spirit. If you take care of it, your body can take care of whatever you want to reach, with power and strength and energy and vitality. You will get there.

He who has health has hope, and he who has hope, has everything.
Arabian Proverb

Love   Live   Laugh

Table of Contents

Love   Live   Laugh

Love   Live   Laugh

Introduction

On July 8, 2011, CNBC broadcast a program during which it was stated that twenty to twenty-five thousand U.S. citizens die every year from medicinal overdose. It is clear that medicine consumption is often the only solution for relieving pain and maintaining reasonably good health. But two of today's well-known facts are that medication costs are rising, and all medicines have side effects. My objective in writing this book is simple: To provide alternatives to medication for solving health-related issues. Some alternatives are as simple as diet and nutrition, stress-reduction, a positive outlook, even a friendly game of Bridge. Another is exercise.

It is my belief that there is a key element overlooked in the treatment of pain and the maintenance of good health—muscles! Muscles support our body's entire structure, so it stands to reason that medicinal relief without building muscles will only be temporary. Exercise is where we find a long-term cure.

Improving the flexibility of muscles remains essential for keeping all parts of our body functional and in good condition. Exercise strengthens muscles, joints, and ligaments. Cardiovascular and respiratory exercises help transport oxygen to all parts of the body, thus improving cell and organ function. Enhanced heart and lung functions help maintain blood pressure and heart rate, and keep blood sugar and cholesterol within proper range. As body tissue receives oxygen and nutrients, you will experience less fatigue and shortness of breath, your sleeping habits will improve, and you will notice a reduction in stress and an increase in energy.

As your body reacts to the positive physiological benefits of exercise, work in healthy eating habits along with logical and positive thinking, and you will not only feel a remarkable overall sense of well-being—you will achieve happiness in all aspects of your life. Good health is a gift, and you can have it when you work for it. We all wish to live longer healthier lives.

Love   Live   Laugh

But we eventually get caught in the same dilemma: How can we afford to live a long life when our capacity to pay high medical costs keeps on depleting? My answer is: We need to manage our own health with a positive outlook and regular exercise. Just thirty minutes a day of low to moderate physical activity can result in all of us living longer, staying healthier, and reducing our healthcare costs.

About My Philosophy

I strongly believe in the motto of the Bill and Melinda Gates Foundation: *All living people need a chance to lead a healthy and productive life*. This book strives towards this objective. Your health depends upon your happiness, and your happiness depends upon your health. When good health and happiness are achieved, you will feel less stress. Less stress leads to rejuvenation of the "brain-engine" of your body.

Your brain is that voice that tells you it's time for a lifestyle change. Your joints ache, you feel tired, you eat the foods that are easiest to acquire—even though they are loaded with fat and calories your body doesn't need—and you find dozens of reasons every day to avoid a new beginning. The most basic first step in practicing better, healthier habits, is simply moving your body. The obstacle to overcome is in your own mind. You must want to try. You must recognize that there are aspects of life you cannot control, but your health doesn't have to be one of them. You must have the desire to live a healthier, happier life. This mindset is rooted in humility.

The lessons expressed in *Healthy Happy You* are similar to the teachings of many great scholarly leaders.

Love   Live   Laugh

Dr. Robindranath Tagore

Dr. Tagore was the 1913 Nobel Prize winner in Literature who reminds us *"The place of prayer is temple."* Expounding upon that statement, he gave us the following philosophies:

Go not to the temple to put flowers upon the feet of God.
First fill your own house with the fragrance of **LOVE.**

Go not to the temple to light candles before the altar of God.
First remove the **darkness of sins from your heart**.

Go not to the temple to bow down your head in prayer.
First learn to bow in **humility** before your **fellow men**.

Go not to the temple to pray on bended knees.
First bend down to **lift someone** who is **<u>downtrodden</u>**.

Go not to the temple to ask for forgiveness for your sins.
First **forgive from your heart those who have sinned** against you.

Buddha

*True knowledge does not come from **religious rituals** but comes from **universe within us**. Such trust gives nirvana to us*, Buddha says. **Meditation controls our body functions, transacts our consciousness, and controls our mind. Deep knowledge** does not come from masters but **comes by mastering**.

Buddha tried deep depreciation and went through considerable hardship and pain, neglecting his desires of material things and moiling his ignorance, vaguer, anger, and jealousy to calm his mind to a sense of peace.

Love   Live   Laugh

He considered life beautiful. He conquered his desires and greed. He expressed himself as a solution of human sufferings without any commandments. His message was:

*See and feel **enlightenment in yourself** when you **comprehend feelings** of others. For you **to be happy others have to be happy** otherwise you can't stay happy. **Turn all greed, anger, and ignorance to love and knowledge**. This **will bring ecstasy** to you.*

Mahatma Gandhi

Indian civil rights leader and pacifist of the early 1900s, Gandhi provides us with these principles:

- Happiness is when and what you **think, say, and do are in harmony**.
- To give **service to a single heart by a single act is better** than thousands of heads bowing in prayer.
- Do not lose faith in humanity. **Humanity is an ocean**. If a few drops of the ocean are dirty, the ocean does not become dirty.

He believes in:

- Seeing a **smile** on faces around you.
- **Achieving** the impossible.
- Showing **love** and **care** to others.
- Giving a **helping hand** to others in their needs.
- Helping others to **enhance their future**.

Love   Live   Laugh

- Being **proud of yourself** in doing such deeds.

Maintaining health is a matter of common sense that depends upon you. Pay attention to a few important aspects. This book will explain how.

Breathing and meditation techniques always help the body to function efficiently and reduce stress. Mental stress reduction allows you to think positively and change your perspective and bring happiness into your life.

1. Manage a healthy diet and add a few daily exercises to control your cholesterol and blood pressure levels. Your body will become shapely and flexible, and give you a refreshing sense of alertness.

2. An active brain requires stimulation, stress reduction, and positivity. Not only will this have an effect on your body's muscles, you will increase your happiness, improve your memory, and give you more power to analyze your surroundings.

3. Believe in your feelings and in yourself to boost your self-confidence and fill you with courage.

4. Rest your body to regenerate body cells and to feel energetic and fit.

5. Reducing body aches and discomfort is a continuous process as you age. The exercises of this book will help to keep your muscles flexible and strong reducing your muscle or joint pain.

My Mission

After my retirement from IBM in 1996, my wife encouraged me to develop my talents and passions in a way that would not only satisfy me, but serve my community as well. "Helping others" is a rather broad challenge, however, and I found that my own definition of connecting with other people frequently changed shape. Regardless, the idea rattled around in my mind for a long time. Like many retirees, I considered a wide variety of options including joining community organizations such as the Red Cross or working in a hospital. Eventually, I realized that my knowledge and experience with human psychology and physiology would be difficult to share with these organizations without a related certification or degree.

Little by little my dream to serve others in a unique way materialized. I learned the different aspects of defining and reducing stress, and I studied the many physical and emotional ways human beings develop healthy and happy ways of life. I practiced methods of expressing positivity and analyzed the results of optimism. Like many health-conscious people, I applied the fundamentals and reaped the benefits of exercise and stretching, but it was important to me to understand, and be able to relate to others, the precise physiological and psychological effects of exercise on a person's mind and body.

My learning curve consisted of immersing myself in information about nutrition and diet management, positivity, massage, brain and memory features as well as arthritic stretches and other exercises. Additionally, I updated and revised what I already knew about breathing and meditation. Over time, I reached the level of a personal trainer.

Throughout my research and learning, I noted positive outcomes at every turn. My excitement and enthusiasm grew and motivated me to revisit avenues for sharing this information in ways that would help others. I began conducting classes on meditation and breathing; stress-free healthy and happy living; and the game of playing bridge (which I have found to stimulate brain power, awareness, and memorization) at beginner, intermediate, and advanced levels.

Love   Live   Laugh

As I observed the responses from class participants, it was soon clear that what I had in my hands was not just another physical fitness program or self-help course. The undeniable link between one's psychological health and one's physical well-being was an aspect of life people desperately wanted to explore and nurture. The stresses of today's world had given birth to an environment in which people of all shapes, sizes, ages, and capabilities sought simple ways to attain health and happiness. Unfortunately and for a variety of reasons, these same people are often reluctant to seek help until problems of mind and body grow to be severe. Thanks to valuable insight from my wife, Meena, who pinpointed a solution—*Healthy Happy You.* A book would help a larger population remove stress, attain happiness, and maintain or improve personal health.

I have written this book with you in mind—your physical condition as well as your state of mind. Good health and a sound mind are our greatest assets. Healthy living reduces dependence on expensive medications and modern medical procedures. Increased vitality affects your ability to think positively and this high-powered combination will enhance your total health beyond your imagination.

Good health is a gift, and you can have it when you work for it. We all wish to live longer, healthier lives. But we get caught in the dilemma of how to afford to live a long life with our capacity to pay high medical costs continually depleting. We have no choice but to manage our own health and take measures to reduce healthcare expenses.

The basic aim of this book, and my sincere desire, is to encourage you to achieve a stress-free, healthy, happy, prosperous life, and at the same time, help you control your escalating healthcare costs. This book shows you how meditation, breathing, and positivity along with stretching and exercise will improve your mental and physical health, and your quality of life in a much broader sense.

Love   Live   Laugh

About This Book

The information in this book comes from my knowledge and experience helping others. I applied every stretch, pose, exercise, and concept to myself. I am not a medical doctor. I have used the *Mayo Clinic Family Health* book for accurate explanations, as it is a valuable source of medical research and medical reasoning. Analytically logical explanations, however, are based upon my own experience, but it is important to note that physical fitness as a whole depends upon an individual's genealogical string and physique. Not every suggestion will apply to you. In such cases, I recommend that you seek the help and advice of your physician.

The explanations in *Healthy Happy You* are general and applicable to most of us. It is common knowledge, after all, that we can live healthy lives by staying active and avoiding smoking, drinking, and junk food. Additional assertions are collected from many other reliable and published medical and psychiatric articles. My goal has been to consolidate this information into a simplistic form for your easy understanding. All of these activities are intended to encourage you and to help you achieve a healthy and happy lifestyle. Every exercise has been tested and validated by many people who have come to my classes for help and who experienced phenomenal success. Your challenge is to apply this information to your health improvement program.

This book is organized into four simple sections.

Section 1 goes behind the scenes into the mental and emotional states that affect your ability and willingness to seek a stress-free healthy life. This section covers maintaining your health with positive thinking; living a happier life by socializing; considerations of diet management and nutrition;

Love   Live   Laugh

simple toning of muscles; stretching and walking in the morning; relaxing and feeling stress-free; and some success stories for encouragement. A study by the World Health Organization many years ago predicted that $604 billion dollars would be used to help Alzheimer sufferers in 2010. This cost is now projected to rise eight-five percent by 2030. For this reason, I included a chapter about stimulating and rejuvenating the brain and enhancing your memory. Think of this entire section as the fundamental building blocks for a healthy life, achieving happiness, and overcoming Alzheimer's disease.

Section 2 delves into the scientific understanding of the physiology of a human body. This includes aerobic and muscular exercises for maintaining and strengthening your body muscles; eye exercises for strengthening eye muscles; therapeutic breathing exercises to strengthen your lungs; abdominal and oblique exercises to keep your body shapely; and how massage helps relax your muscles.

Section 3 presents unique exercises for reducing muscle and joint stiffness, aches, and pains. *Pay careful attention to the precautionary tips to follow when practicing these exercises.* Focus areas include the neck, shoulders, spine, lower back, and knees. This section also touches on avoiding the discomfort of allergies and using meditation to reduce stress and correct sleep disorders. Arthritis is of particular concern to me, which is why I have included a chapter devoted to stretches and massages structured to decrease joint pain. For my own arthritic pain, my doctor told me that I had to learn to live with it. I disagree! Pain is something you do not have to live with or endure.

Section 4 takes certain exercises back to the gym. I've even included a weekly exercise program to get you started.

Love   Live   Laugh

Exercise and Pain

It is my experience that pain management can be accomplished without the use of medication. Most medicines and treatments usually provide temporary relief. The exercises described in this book are meant to manage primarily muscular pain that occurs due to aging or overstressing. Regular activity, such as household chores, will keep muscles flexible, strong, and healthy over the course of your life. However, as you grow older, it becomes necessary to make a few changes in your lifestyle by adding extra stretches and muscle exercises in order to overcome pain and even extend your lifespan. The stretches I describe will present a feeling of light muscular pain as you get started, but you will begin to build muscle mass as you continue with the exercises. Stick with it and you can secure faster or earlier relief—and possibly a permanent cure. Becoming well-informed will help you control your health defensively and slow the aging process.

All exercises should be performed according to your individual physique. Lifting weights might be perfectly appropriate for one person, whereas water aerobics might be better suited for someone experiencing stress on leg and knee joints. Some Tai Chi and yoga exercises have also achieved successful pain relief. But everybody reacts differently and all yoga exercises may not be right for you. Yoga exercises are advertised as panacea for all health and disease problems, but it may not be so.

As with any fitness regimen, your acceptance of these guidelines and your decision to implement them depends upon your personal tolerance level and the advice of a physician who is trained to determine the cause of your discomfort. Like Tai Chi and Yoga, the exercises in this book are believed to work most of the time, but sometimes you need a different approach. When improvement becomes imminent, I recommend that you stay with the selected program to gain a complete cure. In fact, some exercises may specifically require you to continue for a designated length of time in order to achieve meaningful results. It is my hope that you will follow those instructions.

I believe that it is not important to do all of the exercises on a daily basis, but you will find it advantageous to exercise different parts of the body, regularly, on different days. Make sure that over a week time frame, all body muscles are stretched or exercised. It is a physiological fundamental that stretching and exercising are the means to building muscles surrounding a painful region of the body, but you should be aware that building muscles takes time. Do not expect instantaneous relief. Develop patience to endure some discomfort as you proceed.

The exercises and techniques described in this book are the result of twenty years of practice. My assertion is that by maintaining a stress-free healthy life, a person can more easily and quickly overcome the physical and emotional pitfalls that occur every day. Don't underestimate the power of rest! That short nap you feel guilty indulging in during the middle of a day is called a "power nap" by much of today's population. A power nap rejuvenates your body with relaxation. In general, a nap should not exceed thirty minutes since longer naps may upset your system and you may develop a lazy feeling or a headache. Power napping is a fabulous way to recoup your energy. After a power nap you will feel more energetic and healthy. Your body will recover from muscular pains if your nervous system and spinal cord are healthy.

In summary, this book is a compilation of candid advice and meaningful steps to help you understand your physical composition; manage physiological functions such as cholesterol, blood pressure, sugar levels, and oxygen intake; give attention to diet and nutrition; decrease your need for medications and tests; and rejuvenate your senses. Develop a health management plan according to your individual needs and your physical condition. Make it a plan that will motivate you and keep you moving

Love   Live   Laugh

toward your established goals. Always seek the help and advice of your physician.

Finally, have fun! A humorous environment (including practical jokes) is proven to help heal wounds and reduce pain faster than any medication.

REMINDER: If you get dizzy during any exercise, <u>STOP</u> that exercise and consult your physician for recommendations.

Research and Acknowledgments

Healthy Happy You is first and foremost the result of my own passion for helping others find happiness through physical fitness and lasting peace. However, a number of reliable sources and their own research played a significant part in the explanations within the pages of this book. Some of the research is as follows:

Dr. Leigh F. Callahan, Ph.D., director of the Thurston Arthritis Research Center's methodology at the University of North Carolina's orthopedics and social medicine section of the Department of Medicine mentioned on National Public Radio that her research shows that exercise can help a person suffering from arthritic pain.

Washington University in St. Louis declared that their research showed that females who exercise consistently between the ages of 12 and 35 have 23% lower risk of pre-menopausal breast cancer.

The American Academy of Orthopedic Surgeons website www.aaos.org states that exercising your muscles helps you move about more easily by keeping your joints, tendons, and ligaments more flexible. You should engage in weight-bearing exercises, selecting weights in a range suitable for your body.

The *Mayo Clinic Family Health* book explains how different joint muscles may get stressed and cause muscular stresses or body pains. Over-stretching may cause ligament stress.

CIGNA Wellaware for Better Health suggests that exercise is important to have strong muscles so that your lungs don't have to work as hard to supply oxygen to them. Exercise routine plans and activities boost both your muscle strength and lung and heart fitness.

Love   Live   Laugh

Barbara Walters relayed a program on ABC on 4/1/2008 regarding aging and longevity of life. She pointed out that exercises, proper rest, and diets are the three main factors that help enable longevity. (In my opinion two additional factors, stress reduction and the stimulation of the brain could be supplemented to her program. These factors are essential for our healthy living.) Specifically, her program pointed out that protein in our body controls the aging process. Restricting intake of calories helps improve life. A 30% reduction in calories increases longevity by approximately 30%. The key is weight management by dietary consumption of oils, greens, meats, and fruits. Maintaining healthy weight keeps blood pressure, blood glucose, triglycerides and cholesterol at an acceptable level.

The University of Kansas published a report stating that regular exercises may help slow the progress of Alzheimer disease. Researchers focused on brain atrophy caused by Alzheimer and used MRI scans to measure patients' brains. Patients who were physically active were found to suffer less brain shrinkage than their counterparts.

My Gratitude

This book reflects my own knowledge and learning, but also the help of many of my friends—including my physician friends. I especially thank my father who initiated this interest in me.

After my retirement from IBM as an engineer, I focused my attention on exercises, human psychology, and the human physique. To gain this level of knowledge, I educated myself to the level of a personal trainer, read material on human physiology and psychology, explored diet management schemes, practiced positivity, and examined approaches for staying healthy. I used the stretches—and created some of my own—to develop relationships between physiology and muscular exercise. Without such experimentation, research, and understanding, I could not have written this book.

Love   Live   Laugh

My very close friend, **Mr. Jagdish Saran Agrawal**, a writer, speaker, entrepreneur and CEO, helped me develop this book at all stages. With his creative mind, knowledge, and guidance, I am able to reach this level of publication. He was always ready to help me. I am very much obliged to him.

I thank **Dr. Van K. Tharp**, a writer, speaker, entrepreneur and president of the International Institute of Trading and Mastering (also known as Tharp Trading and Mastering), for his advice and ideas that made me look deeper into the subject I was exploring. I revised the material many times as I went along. His help made me reach my objectives. I thank him for his help.

Dr. Vasishtha Majmundar, MD—a surgeon and anesthesiologist—reviewed the book for its medical references and medical terminology. His advice and help in numerous ways made the book easier to understand. I thank him for his help.

Dr. Raj Makam, MD, M.R.C.P., F.A.C.P.—a gastroenterologist—gave me valuable input. His support and his reorganization of this material helped define this book's topics. He added medical clarity to the book. His help encouraged me to accomplish my dream. I personally thank him for his effort and help.

Janice Stolzenberg, a student of many of my classes and a great motivator who speaks very highly of my research and results, helped to promote my Breathing and Meditation class. Through her input, my class was featured on the local evening news program in 2009. I credit her interview with helping bring success to the program. She increased my confidence and made the material worth an ABC news program. I sincerely appreciate her help and thank her for all her efforts.

On a personal level, I must thank my daughter, **Tuhina Ruff**, who uncompromisingly supported me. She reviewed this book multiple times to give it a form and a shape. Without her loving hands I would have been handicapped to complete this work. She is a regular attendee of a health club. She understands the basics and the details of many exercises. Her background was extremely valuable to me, including her engineering and M.B.A. degrees, along with her experience as a community treasurer, a local school helper, and the mother of three beautiful children.

My deepest thanks go to all others who helped me and who contributed to this book including Richard Timothy Ruff.

Scope of this Book

The message conveyed by *Healthy Happy You* can be expressed through these   thirteen focus areas, which are discussed in detail in the pages of this book.

1. Use meditation techniques to enhance your life.

2. Enjoy a stress-free, healthy, and happy life.

3. Live with energy, enthusiasm, and empathy.

4. Fulfill the purpose of your life by socializing.

5. Achieve ultimate happiness.

6. Look for positivity and goodness in others.

7. Live a life with positive outlook.

8. Overcome body pains and aches without medications.

9. Tone body muscles with activities.

10. Stimulate your brain and memory.

11. Distance yourself from sorrows.

12. Manage your diet with healthy foods.

13. Reduce escalating health costs.

Love   Live   Laugh

Healthy Life

Healthy living depends upon many factors; most of them are within our control. These factors include positive thinking, staying active, managing diet, eating healthy foods, maintaining the health of your brain, strengthening your lungs via breathing techniques, reducing stress through meditation, and keeping your body flexible and healthy by stretching and exercising. Apply these disciplines depends upon your physique. Handle only what your physique allows you. Make sure that your planned activity is approved.

"All growth depends upon activity. There is no development physically or intellectually without effort, and effort means work."
Calvin Coolidge

Whatever your plan is, accept it whole-heartedly with self-reliance and self-confidence. Make a resolution for yourself that you will stick to your plan without hesitation. Your commitment will help you avoid procrastination and the associated hardship. Create a perception of yourself since your perceptions will portray your looks. Develop your mental state to look at positive aspects all the time and under all circumstances.

"Character is built daily by the way one thinks and acts, thought by thought, action by action." *Helen Douglas*

Newton's Law states, "There is an equal and opposite reaction to every action." This applies in many different ways. It means that your

Love   Live   Laugh

actions and efforts are reactionary. With positive thinking, good occurrences happen and vice versa.

Achieve Ultimate Happiness

"Life is 10 percent what you make it, and 90 percent how you make it." Irving Berlin

Happiness is a state of mind that overcomes your stress. Happiness appears in different forms in our lives. Happiness can be characterized as temporary happiness or it can be a long-term happiness. Temporary happiness is related to more self-indulgence; examples are buying or acquiring things. After fulfillment of the initial desire, you may find emptiness.

Long-term happiness is self-gratifying and selfless. Happiness due to self-gratification comes from within when you are successful in your actions. When you are not trying to satisfy your own ego, selfless happiness will emerge. It is happiness due to no reason at all.

Nature brings about happiness by staying positive in all circumstances and at all times. It directs your mental state toward your positive outlook. It is your thinking that will lead you to search for and see goodness in others. It involves training of your mind and your actions and statements.

Enjoy Stress-free, Healthy and Happy Life *(refer chapter: Happiness & Socializing)*

All your successful resolutions will power you with self-strength and self-satisfaction. Understand and develop your interests.

Love   Live   Laugh

"Chance favors those in motion." James H. Austin

When you have not planned well, the achievement of your objectives becomes difficult. When the situation is not corrected, procrastination may set in and your senses deprive of optimism, thus causing your goals to slide.

Learn the techniques that are related to your genealogy and organize yourself to make them easy for you to follow. Consistent practice will be the foundation of your self-confidence. It will increase your energy level and that will encourage you to continue with your program.

Live with Energy, Enthusiasm, and Empathy

"The world belongs to the energetic." Ralph Waldo Emerson

Your health will improve with enthusiastic activities and you will sleep better. Keep your optimism to achieve your healthy objectives. Self-commitment and self-determination to achieve a goal will keep your body in a healthy condition for the rest of your life.

Fulfill the Purpose of Your Life

"The great use of life is to spend it doing something that will outlast it." William James

Looking ahead to your healthy living should generate optimism and self-esteem. Self-confidence and faith are essential parts of developing optimism and a feeling of being healthy. Achievements will encourage your confidence level and your positive outlook.

Love   Live   Laugh

The premise of this book depends upon your consistent analysis and improvement with a healthy state of mind.

A British saying is, "A friend in need is a friend indeed." Consider this book a friend that gives you an opportunity to follow the principles of stress-free healthy living.

Gerald F. Seib once wrote in a *Wall Street Journal* article that President Ronald Reagan used to tell a story of an optimistic young boy. The boy's optimism would allow him to see gold in a barrel of dirt. The moral of the story was, "You need to have optimism before reaching your goal."

Analyze all your planned actions carefully to achieve your goal. Optimism and faith will result in self-confidence for a healthy life. Your selection of choices depends upon your knowledge, experience, and background. Let this book help you with your plans.

"Look deep into nature, and then you will understand everything better." Albert Einstein

Distance Yourself from Sorrows *(refer chapter: 'Resting & Being Stress-free')*

"We either make ourselves miserable or we make ourselves strong. The amount of work is the same." Carlos Castenada

Human nature, in general, seeks to reduce stress, daily inconveniences, and body aches. You may like to seek some prescription drug since it is an easy route, but natural cures, for the most part, have no side effects. You should lean toward finding a natural cure as often as possible.

Love   Live   Laugh

Evaluate your tolerance to bear some discomfort without medicinal treatment. Compare the benefits of a natural cure versus a medicinal cure. In some cases, you may have to use medicine(s) during your evaluation period.

Overcome your Body Discomforts and Aches *(refer section 3)*

This book will help you recover from many muscular pains through natural means. The exercises I describe will strengthen your muscles to help the body overcome from aches. Remember, natural processes require a longer time to recoup and to rebuild your muscles to feel comfortable.

Small successes are parts of your bigger success. Keep your full faith and optimism in your success by continuous practicing without skepticism.

"Better do in inches than in yards." Chinese Proverb

Yoga developed a laughing exercise, called "Laughter Yoga," to keep you healthy and happy. You may wonder, why laugh for no reason? Jeanette, a student in my "Healthy Living" class told me that "Laughter Yoga" helped reduce her arthritic pains. A habit of laughing will keep you happier with a smile on your face.

Children, in general, get lots of exercise from their daily activities by playing outside with their friends. It is not mandatory for them to do any special exercise unless their body requires it. Children exercise in many different ways—by biking or by running around or playing other physical games. If someone has health problems due to a lack of outdoor activity or dieting, he/she will need help. Indulging in food or in computer games are non-physical activities. Children should be encouraged to play in fresh air, rather than be monotonous, so that they stay healthy.

Love   Live   Laugh

Meditate to reduce Mental Stress *(refer chapter: 'Meditation Techniques')*

A Sanskrit mantra states: "Yogah Karmasu Kaushalam."

This verse means "Yoga as a part of your daily life will bring success in all of your actions and ventures." The mantra provides not only physiological and psychological help but guides you through the proven ways to overall success in your actions and enterprises.

Reduce Your Escalating Health Costs

"Practice makes a man perfect."

"Nothing ventured, nothing gained or lost except an opportunity"

Swami

A swami is a holy person in India who has acquired, with practice, nature's knowledge. He learned these techniques from his Guru who is also a Swami. "Swami" in Sanskrit implies:

"He who knows and is master of himself"

"Owner of oneself"

"Believer of Natural Cures and Nature's ways"

"He who is a scholar and master of certain practice of Vendata"

"He who is Free from the senses"

Swami means "a master" – mastery over oneself, so that his internal self shines through. Swami sets aside limits to his worldly pursuits and achieves the highest spiritual realization. He services others selflessly.

Swami does not claim allegiance to any particular group or religion, and sees all as the outpouring of one, invisible reality, truth or God, the absolute reality. Swami gives up his personal identity, including nationality or family identities. His identity relates to perception for the benefit of others whom he serves. He indulges to achieve benefits for the world. He attains a universal love.

The qualities of the swami are attained with lots of practice and self-dedication under the supervision of his Guru. He attains elusive qualities to inspire others and his followers to achieve an Absolute Reality in the world.

This book, *Healthy Happy You*, will help you to acquire similar qualities as a swami. It will help you to learn and apply positive evaluations and thinking, breathing and meditation actions, and to overcome many diseases, and acquire peace of mind and righteous decisions and actions

Love   Live   Laugh

under all circumstances. Such actions will lead you to achieve true happiness in your life and maintain your good health and high spirit.

Section 1: Body Stimuli

Chapter 1

Positivity & Happiness

Steve attended my "Healthy Happy Living" class and wanted to know my ideas on positive thinking. I responded that we are all humans. We get easily attracted to negative thoughts and adapt them because they are exciting and give us a lot to talk about. A perfect example of this is how negativity attracts the news media. Bad news often is the exciting news and that helps their sale. The problem is that negative thoughts breed negative feelings. Our mental reasoning gets distorted with the negative analysis. This leads to negative expression.

What does an overall sense of negativity bring to us? Steve and I agreed that it generates negative thoughts, sadness, worry, and stress. We think unkind thoughts about others that may manifest in our power to invite negative actions. If we consciously think and analyze, we may question ourselves. Does this kind of thinking lead us to any benefit? The answer to this question is obviously "No." Such thoughts lead us toward nothing but terrorizing others and ourselves. Our goal should be to try to avoid such circumstances.

As humans, we are continually faced with two choices: Think negatively or think positively. Having already described the results of negative thinking, I suggested to Steve that look what positivity brings.

Simply put, positive thoughts breed good feelings within us and enhance our faith in our fellow human beings. It brings about courage, objectivity, and healthy actions encouraging us to help others. It also nurtures in each of us a feeling of self-confidence, self-esteem, and faith in this world. Positivity is what enables us to live stress-free and peacefully in our society. We judge others not by their looks but by their deeds.

Love   Live   Laugh

After this explanation, Steve asked the most important question. How do you achieve the path of positivity? My answer was *practice*. It takes a lot of practice to recognize positive qualities, dedicate yourself to the idea, and overlook the negative thoughts and tendencies that will try to creep in. Adopting a sense of positivity, however, will change your character.

Difficulties are things that show a man's nature - Epictelus

Meditation is one means to overcoming negativity and helping you convert your thoughts toward positivity. Changing the thinking process requires a great deal of concerted effort in training of the brain. You will become optimistic after you replace all negative interpretations with positive interpretations and see the results. This change comes from personal actions and dedication to the change.

- The first step is to remove yourself from negative surroundings.
- The second step is to avoid or reject negative ideas.
- The third step is to determine the objective of a message before jumping to a conclusion.
- The fourth step is to determine the positive side of the message.

These four simple actions will surround you with positive energy. Once you attain this level, you will attain charismatic happiness. People around you will notice—you will have a happier look on your face from your positive outlook on life!

"So how exactly do you "think positively?"

Love   Live   Laugh

Whenever you hear news or observe an event, your first thought should be to determine what is the goodness in the message, rather than what is bad news in the message. With consistent practice, you will eventually only look for the positive side of events. You will develop a habit of seeing only goodness and you will ignore or overlook negativity without giving it a second thought or wasting your energy on it.

The process of positive thinking will eventually become part of your life and you will be able to honestly label yourself a *positive thinker*. We all have at least one positive quality within us. All their energy seems to go toward positive thinking and it is a characteristic that is always on display. When you become a positive thinker, you will influence others to better behavior without trying to transform them.

When you weigh the benefits of positivity, you will develop faith in your thinking and your actions. You will demonstrate self-esteem and self-confidence. Others will believe in you not only by your statements, but by your actions. Emotional energy developed by positive thinking energizes you to get over your anger. It will give you flexibility that reduces your illnesses. When you have down days, it may be time to keep a low profile. Always evaluate your thoughts first before speaking out.

Create a belief deep within you and recognize that nothing is yours or mine in this world. Everything, whether finite or infinite, belongs to the universe. Your conscious and unconscious thoughts will naturally lead your life toward happiness. It is a fundamental desire of every living creature. After all, we are part of and belong to this universe, too. Ours is a universe that is made up of five elements—space, wind, fire, water, and the earth. Individually, we may try to divide these elements, but it is virtually impossible to do so.

In my discussion with Steve, I summarized the principles of positivity in this way. Recognize that all good thoughts tend to occur according to your wishes. You will use less physical and emotional energy since you are not

Love   Live   Laugh

stressed and since you do not have to worry about the final results. Why? Because positive ideas bring about positive results for you. Positive results continuously generate more positive thoughts. This infusion of positivity will enhance your life. Therefore, positive thinking becomes a key to your happiness.

Have you noticed that happy people smile a lot and they look fresher? Good things happen to make us happy, that gives us more to smile about and us feel relaxed and calm. Our every message should relay some positive aspect in us. You will realize that on the occasion when you do not have anything good to say, you will choose not to say anything at all. You will naturally begin to only send messages—whether verbal or nonverbal—that relay the positivity that has become a part of you.

Steve asked me, "Do we have to find an excuse for our happiness?"

My answer: "No."

To elaborate, I explained that caring for others is a joy that represents our love to others. Happiness is not something you find, it is what you create. Learn to enjoy your life by finding inner smiles. Become more receptive to positive ideas that will lead you toward goodness in your life.

Positivity lets you lead a happy and healthy life since your stress is minimized and your relaxation gives you extra energy. During the relaxed periods you will find additional time to contemplate more good thoughts that will fill your heart with smiles. This is the reason why when you meet a swami, your first impression is a positive one and your attention is drawn to his smiling face. (Swamis are carefree persons who enjoy the gifts given by the nature of positive thinking.) Joy, happiness, excitement, and contentment may even help individuals with cardiovascular diseases.

Love   Live   Laugh

I told Steve that I thought Jesus Christ probably always had a smile on his face. "After all," as I explained, "Jesus said, 'Love thy neighbor.'" These three words say it all. Of course, his is a theological statement, but there is a lot of meaning attached to it. For Steve's benefit, I tried to analyze Jesus' <u>words</u> philosophically, the way I see it.

First, *who is thy neighbor?*

A neighbor is a general human with whom you commonly associate or deal with or who surrounds you in your environment.

What does Jesus mean by *love?*

Philosophically, I interpret love as a positive feeling in your heart for others. For example, if you think negatively about another person you will not be enamored with that person. You will not be able to show love to that person. If, however, you recognize positive qualities in that other person, you will find it easy, and natural, to let your love flow through you to your neighbor. Without positivity, love is not possible. As your own positivity grows within you, you can develop even deeper feelings. So you see, without positive thinking and a deep-rooted sense of happiness, these three words of Jesus Christ, 'love thy neighbor,' are relatively meaningless.

Let me use my father as another example. My father once said, "Listen to everyone and do what you consider is right." A person with negative thinking may interpret this statement as a selfish statement. With negative thinking, one may interpret it as a suggestion to ignore everybody's ideas and do whatever you like. On the other hand, with my positive interpretation I believe he desired that I weigh the different ideas and suggestions set before me prior to embarking on my selection. In other words, I should wisely analyze the collection of ideas and select the one that is the best of them all. See how you can interpret the same statement

Love   Live   Laugh

differently depending upon your own mental state? A negative thought will lead you to interpret such a statement negatively while positive thinking will lead you to interpret it positively.

Peace, joy, and happiness in our lives come from our becoming selfless, honest, and servants to others without looking for any reward. In addition, you develop your own strength by believing in yourself. I asked Steve to consider this statement: *"With my positive thinking I am proud of what I am, who I am, and I am peaceful"*. I added that you couldn't just say these words; you must *feel* them, along with the joy and happiness of your life.

Your life is what you make it to be. Self-respect and self-esteem are what enables you to pursue your passions and accomplishments.

Do not acquire anger, greed, or self-desires.
Acquire peace and happiness.

Follow this statement and you will experience a higher level of self-esteem. Your thoughts and approach to life will become flexible and will flourish happiness within you.

Happiness will get rid of a sparse diet of promises and excuses for the implementation of good ideas. Excuses spread like a virus and must be eliminated. Avoid procrastination and you will sow a seed of happiness that will lead to good health and positive outcomes.

You can master your own mind. Learn to accept your environment as it is by distinguishing good ideas from bad and judging right from wrong. When new ideas come to you, implement them within a reasonable period. If you wait, circumstances may change and you might miss your chance. Such a "failure" (in one sense of the word) will leave you dissatisfied and unhappy.

Love   Live   Laugh

Be flexible! Flexibility teaches us that by embracing our failures and frustrations, we give ourselves permission to be human. This is like therapy—we allow ourselves to be more open to our positive emotions and our emotions help us to think in a more positive manner. Flexibility will enhance our happiness.

Maintaining good health is an important key to our happiness. Happiness is based on the satisfaction of our desires while unhappiness is a result of excessive desires. Alongside desires you should have aspirations. While both desires and aspirations are essential in life, you must set a limit according to your capacity. Develop a habit of accepting trouble gracefully while still trying to achieve or accomplish your goals.

Achieving happiness through contentment, reduced mental stress, and anxiety are the best ways to develop self-esteem and decision making ability.

One who is calmer, relaxed, and outgoing will have an active social life without developing dementia.

Analyze all situations with a positive outlook help change the terms of love.

Nearly a dozen studies have shown that positive thinking makes people contented, happier, and live healthier and longer lives. A happy person is less likely to suffer from heart attacks, strokes, and rheumatoid arthritis. Psychology department research from Carnegie Mellon and the University of Pennsylvania points to a single finding: *People who express positive emotions suffer less compared to those who express negative*

Love   Live   Laugh

emotions, including anger, sadness, or stress. The research involved was directed to the subjects' immune systems that might have adverse effects under the stress conditions. Studies at other universities pointed to different immune proteins that also grew under happier circumstances. The combination of this research supports the suggestion that 'happier people live healthier and longer.' In fact, experts who are positive psycho-sociologists have found that the simple act of being grateful for what you have can help improve your outlook in life and bring you happiness. Try to remember to relate all of life's events and circumstances with respect to positivity. In essence, you should reject negative events.

To achieve this level of positivity and happiness, take to heart the following common sense steps:

- Always go for real and attainable goals.

- Think about happiness in terms of leading a meaningful life.

- Accept others and do not evaluate them harshly. Do not expect any return for the good deeds you do. Let the actions of others surprise you.

- Help others by doing good deeds. I define help in this way: *When you help someone, that person benefits from your actions.*

- Make a "gratitude visit" or deliver a thank-you note to those who have been especially kind or helpful to you. You will get pleasure by remembering that positive event of your life. Plus, you may strengthen your relationship with a person who may bring future happiness to you.

- Focus on your accomplishments – count your good deeds of the day. Most people spend more time thinking about what went wrong rather than what went right. Jot down three things that went well in a day then examine the reasons for such success. This exercise will help you

Love   Live   Laugh

feel more grateful of your own character. It will increase your courage and self-esteem.

- Increase your awareness of your ego and get involved to solve crises without feeling lonesome.

Ralph Waldo Emerson wrote, "To laugh often and much; to win the respect of intelligent people and the affection of children; to earn the appreciation of honest critics and endure the betrayal of false friends; to appreciate beauty; to find the best in others; to leave the world a bit better— whether by a healthy child, a garden patch, a redeemed social condition; and to know even one life has breathed easier because of you, you have lived and have succeeded in leading a happy life."

Happy people are they who laugh and have peace of mind.

The Hallmark TV channel showed a program called *The Good Witch* in February of 2009 and repeated it many times later. The woman who acted as the "good witch" always showed her love and smile to others while most of the town was against her. She always had positive emotions even in tough situations. She dealt with the town using her faith and by staying positive she won people over. She earned the respect and appreciation of the whole town. This example of positivity may not be an easy task to accomplish but consistent belief and a positive attitude can win over the world.

The happiest people on this planet are not those who live on their own terms but are those who change their terms for someone they love. What you achieve or become depends upon you, your thoughts, and your beliefs. Your implementations and actions will reflect your thoughts. Your beliefs stimulate the power within you that penetrates into your thoughts. A dynamic attitude and positive thinking are the strong magnetic forces that attract good results. Do not let negativity take over and destroy your ambitions. Mark Twain said, "I had many fears in my life, most of which never happened." Do not be afraid of being positive. You have everything to gain and you will not lose.

A student named Pat told me after one of my classes that she was a very negative person. She went on to admit that my class had taught her how to change herself to become a positive person. She assured me that she would work to attain a positive attitude.

Never doubt the creative power of enthusiasm to achieve reasonable goals.

Human evolution and development depend upon energy. Values and qualities emanate by managing energy.

Positive thinking is a powerful tool; believe it and apply it for your peace, contentment, and happiness. Define yourself with your positive views rather than with your negative views.

Love   Live   Laugh

Chapter 2

Happiness & Socializing

As America's population ages it is faced with questions about longevity and quality of life. To maintain a desirable quality of life, we have to be happy and socialize with our friends, laugh and enjoy our intimacy.

Happiness really depends upon us and our own psychology, our social circle, and our socialization level. As individuals, we can work to improve our environment. Happiness resides within us and is related to many psychological factors. It depends upon how we view and interpret our surroundings. We can look at our world with positivity or negativity. To be healthy, we must select the positive aspects.

Psychology is a science of beliefs. Your beliefs will be based on what suits you or on what you feel. Events that happen become part of the environment in which you live. If you chalk up the results of these events to your beliefs, you are on your way to determining a solution to your psychological beliefs when they need amending for your health and happiness. When your beliefs cost you your health, it is time to make some changes. Take personal responsibility for your beliefs and for your mental state.

Healthy beliefs will give you limitless power to overcome unhappiness. Happiness depends quite a bit upon your expectations. Outcomes that differ from your expectations may be very hard to accept. As I view it, your personal approach and psychology affect how you perceive certain situations as well as how you may react to them.

The idea that happiness leads to good health is no mystery. To achieve good health and stay happy, you need to put effort into resolving unhappy situations. When positive outcomes and happiness result in good health

Love   Live   Laugh

people tend to become more social which, in turn, will continue to increase your happiness level. Sometimes this means forgiving and forgetting misdeeds—both of others and your own. Eternal happiness is yours for the taking when you practice forgiveness and resolve unhappiness.

Experts, who call themselves 'positive-psychologists,' have found that simple acts of gratitude can improve your outlook and bring about happiness and improved health. Let us look at some ways to be accomplishing this.

- Enjoy the company of others. Socialize!

- Set your objectives with love and attention, whatever they may be. Accomplish them with self-confidence and you will be happy with the outcomes.

- Nurture that feeling of self-confidence and believe that you are a worthwhile human being.

- Limit your expectations for your achievements. Otherwise, not achieving all of your objectives will make you unhappy and dissatisfied. All levels of achievement should bring happiness to you.

- Avoid predicaments that will make you unhappy. Believe in your own actions and accept your surroundings.

- Feel the love of others and convey your love to those you encounter. Love is the affinity that links us and draws us together.

- Accept that others appreciate your deeds and respond with gratitude.

- Laugh and enjoy others in a social environment. Laugh a lot to give your mood a lift and make your environment a healthier one.

- Meditate to reduce stress and increase mental peace.

- Eliminate jealousy from your emotions. Develop instead a habit of being genuinely happy and appreciative of others.

Love   Live   Laugh

- Look to the future with a sense of hope. Treat tomorrow as another opportunity to smile and laugh. It will improve your immune system.

- Reach for real, attainable goals and think of being happy in terms of leading a meaningful life.

- Relax and increase your energy by staying positive.

- Do kind deeds without reward.

- Accept your faults when they happen. Laugh them out!

- Take pleasure in the material things you have and enjoy them without wanting more.

These points are all part of our human psychology. How you perceive and react to things are features of your happiness. Your immune system responds to your emotional state. Relaxation significantly improves a body's functions—from the lymph system to the spleen and bone marrow. When your mind and body are in harmony, your behavior will reflect the peace, health, contentment, and happiness in your life. Boost your immune system by strengthening your muscles and laughing! Showing happiness with a consistent smile on your face is the real answer to stress reduction.

Psycho-sociologists believe healthy living comes with happiness. Happiness reduces illnesses. In 2006, Harvard University actually offered a course called "How to Be Happy." The course became the most popular one in their psychology department. Used in the course was Alan Gettis's book, *The Happiness Solution: Finding Joy and Meaning in an Upside Down World* (Goodman Beck Publishing, 2008). This book is a fascinating collection of short stories, myths, and anecdotes that support the idea that happiness is within each of us and it becomes accessible when we seek it.

Happiness comes in different forms, depending on the circumstances. Some instances may last for a short time—let's call this temporary

Love   Live   Laugh

happiness. Temporary happiness is mainly a result of self-indulgence, such as acquiring things. The joy that comes from acquiring something will live as the short-term satisfaction of fulfilling your desire since you will soon start looking for the next item to acquire. Despite our tendency to accumulate things, it is an accepted truth that happiness cannot be achieved through possessions.

True happiness emanates from formless dimensions within us and from our subconscious. Our personal achievements are related to our happiness, but for true selfless satisfaction, look for *happiness for no reason at all*. Make it part of your nature to be happy and stay happy all the time.

At this point in our discussion, Steve asked, "How can someone be happy for no reason at all?"

I explained that the key is to seek happiness for the long haul, not short-term satisfaction. The joy of *being* should be our only true happiness in life. No situation is permanent. We must remain flexible so that we change along with our environment. As I described in Chapter: 'Positivity & Happiness' happiness comes from your positive thoughts and from your mental state. When you seek and find goodness in the actions and statements of others, and within yourself, the positive thinking that results will bring you solace and true happiness.

"But," Steve interjected, "What do you do about the people out there who are led by ignorance and who lose themselves to anger, displeasure, jealousy, prejudice, and other worldly passions?"

My answer is, "There is no such thing as ***mine*** in this world."

To spread the notion of happiness, people must adopt the belief that everything belongs to a natural world. As easily as our surroundings are created by a series of causes and conditions, these same surroundings can—

Love   Live   Laugh

and will—disappear from this world in the same way. The human mind is a creator and a controller of our own destiny and happiness. When you speak or act with your good intentions, happiness will follow you like a shadow. A calm mind invites peacefulness and you will experience happiness day and night without much effort.

Let us consider the big picture. Powerful forces eventually get released within you to generate the desire and create the ability for you to live peacefully and happily in the present state. You learn from your mistakes when you examine them objectively. Such training and thinking will create a constant flow of positive energy within you and will lead you toward hope, confidence, and good will toward others. It's about staying in that flow and becoming completely absorbed in your work or in the pursuit of your goals. Stay involved with people who you love, and socialize and take part in leisure activities and hobbies. Social connections are a vital part of creating that peaceful state of contentment that leads to happiness.

Here's an exercise that you can do anytime and anyplace. Simply visualize happiness. What does it look like to you? How does it feel? Hold that image in your mind and place your full faith in your thoughts and your beliefs. Stop comparing your achievements and activities with others. Do not downplay yourself but instead rejoice in your accomplishments and in the accomplishments of others. Now, see how it works.

This exercise will make your mind calm. You will feel mentally peaceful, like nothing will unduly bother you. While reality and your anxieties may result in a mixture of successes and failures, your peaceful approach will bring you more successes than failures. You will observe that you will never have to doubt this creative power of enthusiasm within you.

Happiness is a result of your recognizing and appreciating all that you have. You generate the power to judge correctly between good and bad, right and wrong, in order to lead an effective life. Looking beyond your horizon awakens you to the newness in your life, and your experiences become the substance of your wisdom, bringing you honor and prosperity.

Here are a few other thoughts for mental stimulation:

- Smile, laugh, and believe that happiness resides within you.
- Control your desires by controlling your temptations.
- Keep your mind away from greed by molding and leaning toward purity.
- Avoid anger by staying away from disputes.
- Remove idleness from your life. It is a waste of time. Bring purpose to your being.
- Practice what you preach to others by setting good examples. Keep yourself faithful to your words.
- Engulf your mind with compassionate feelings.
- Increase your awareness of your ego but solve crises without feeling alone.

Only you can create a state of happiness for yourself. We separate our *needs* from our *wants* depending upon our survival requirements. Showing our appreciation and kindness to others with our actions become a source of enjoyment. It also helps us to be part of our society. Don't be afraid to show your happiness. Let go of that need to show off your position or status to others. Remember what we said about temporary happiness? The fulfillment of wants leads to short-term joy. For permanent happiness, you need to change your attitude and focus on reasonable, attainable expectations. Accept your environmental surroundings, as they exist. If you are unhappy about the present condition, do something to change it.

Love   Live   Laugh

Happiness lies within us.

We all want peace and happiness in our lives. Be a positive thinker, a selfless person, and stay honest. Provide service to others without a reward. You may not immediately see the benefits of your actions but you will be happy by showing your love and empathy to others. One becomes what one thinks and feels. Think and look only to the good qualities in others, not the faults. Consciously getting involved brings about internal prosperity and happiness. Newton's third law of motion states that "for every action there is an equal and opposite reaction." This is now considered a common sense law and is applicable to all different situations. Apply this law to your own dealings. When you show love, care, and appreciation to others, others value your feelings and respond with their respect and appreciation back to you.

Now, all this talk of positive thinking, socialization, and happiness is not to say that at some point in your life you won't feel down, or even depressed. It happens to everyone. You don't, however, have to get stuck in that unhappy feeling. When you begin to feel the symptoms of depression (fatigue, loss of appetite, isolation, loneliness, and despair, to name a few), take the time to concentrate on how you are feeling. Identify the cause, as realistically as possible. Then, determine a solution to resolve the situation, or change the conditions surrounding it.

Here are some specific actions to take, both physical and emotional:

- Identify the cause(s) of your depression.
- Remain optimistic and hope to resolve it.
- Maintain your health.
- Control your emotions and avoid actions that could be in any way dangerous or disastrous.

Love   Live   Laugh

- Reduce unimportant burdensome tasks and relax.

- Stay calm and serene; look only to your future.

- Eliminate resentment toward others. Gather energy from the power of your subconscious mind. This will help you feel more positive, override perceived failures, and help you return to a happier state.

- Visualize a mental image of yourself as the healthy and vigorous person, you are. Let this image inspire you.

Our thought processes lead us to management of our senses. For example, let's say you're experiencing anger and frustration. Your objective is to return to 'peace of mind.' As I mentioned, all your enjoyment depends upon your positive and negative senses. When your good sense is not satisfied, negativity takes over to develop your anger. During an angry period, your thinking power will suffer and your power of understanding will vanish. So, how can you achieve your objective?

To develop 'peace of mind' you need to control your senses by diverting your attention towards positivity and happiness. Your positive sense will help you to judge your objective correctly and weigh the good and the bad, or right and wrong. Continuously remind yourself that you want to be happy. Set a simple goal: To get rid of your preconceived ideas and notions. Then, rearrange your surroundings to help you meet your goal. It's a continual process, but as your mindset changes and your brain begins receiving positive messages, your body will respond with positive feedback as well and you will once again be on your way to a state of happiness.

This problem of depression and peace of mind is often seen in retirees. For some, retirement is a killer. After all, we, and those we know, spend years working. Then one day our focus changes from work and earning a living, to having the time to do the things we love and enjoy. Retirement simply means that no longer have to worry about daily earnings. Be careful

Love   Live   Laugh

not to neglect your mental and physical fitness just because you are now retired. In fact, now is a good time to devote even more time to your health. The work that gave you frustrations and stress is gone from your life.

At the age of 96, Paul played bridge and enjoyed it immensely. He was very slow in his game, but he made good judgments. And, if he made any mistakes, he didn't have to lose sleep over them! I suggest that you engage in a hobby that you enjoy—something that you could not do during your years working your regular job. Now that you are free from that responsibility, you should enjoy your life of retirement. Boredom can kill you. Keep yourself healthy by staying busy.

Accept successes, not failures.
Resolve to strive for and achieve peace of mind.

Love   Live   Laugh

Chapter 3

Diet Management & Healthy Foods

On a break during one my "Healthy Living" classes, a student named Carol confided in me that she is health conscious but concerned about the foods she and her family eat. She has read many articles about healthy food but she finds it difficult to determine which information she can trust. Her goal is for her family to eat nutritious food and stay healthy.

I reminded Carol that although I am not a registered dietitian, I have done considerable research into nutrition and I was happy to share my findings with her. First and foremost, I told her, good health depends upon reducing (or eliminating) the bad habits of eating junk food, smoking, and drinking. I also pointed out that whenever possible, avoid medications—including antibiotics—unless they are deemed essential. As an alternative, she should turn to *probiotics*—the "good bacteria" that helps our intestines and digestion. After all, I said, she and her family will reap the benefits of good food habits for their entire lives.

Defining "Healthy" Foods

Unfortunately, our government has yet to define specifications for what designates "health food" healthy foods and which manufacturers must meet. However, healthier foods are generally defined as those with:

- Limited sodium content
- Minimal total calories
- Reduced saturated fats

Sodium, calories, and fat all can adversely affect a body's blood pressure. Yet, there are plenty of foods on our grocery store shelves that are high in these three elements, and labeled "healthy." In the absence of clear guidelines, we are at the mercy of manufacturers to define "healthy" foods.

Today's media has inundated us with articles, programs, and advertisements about healthy eating. And soon after the word "health food" earned buzzword status, food providers and marketers changed their labels to call their product a "healthy food." Some simply reduced their product's fat content, then added the word "healthy" to its label or packaging. Restaurant food might be full of sodium, calories, and fat, and still be listed as a healthy food as food preparers are more inclined to serve tastier food in order to appeal to their consumers' taste buds. The good news is that soon, restaurant owners will be required to add food ingredients to their menus.

I suggested to Carol that we look at the effect of sodium, calories, and saturated fats present in most of food items. Granted, these three elements are needed somewhat for healthy living, but you must pay attention to the amounts found in food. Read the item label! Judge healthy foods according to their contents. You can't afford not to. Good nutrition guards against disease, obesity, and diabetes.

Sodium

More than 1500-2000mg of sodium intake a day is known to increase the systolic blood pressure that causes a risk of heart disease. High blood pressure presses against the walls of the aorta and arteries and causes swelling of these arteries or dilation of our aorta. Sodium also forces our bodies to retain water, a condition that causes kidney disease. However, our bodies do need a small amount of sodium to control our nerve impulses, relax our muscles, and balance fluids.

The *Wall Street Journal* published an article on January 21, 2010, that suggested that cutting dietary salt could prevent tens of thousands of heart attacks, strokes, and deaths. So where does all this salt come from? Approximately seventy-five percent comes from processed foods. The American Heart Association (AHA) published new guidelines to reduce the daily intake of sodium to no more than 1500-2000mg a day.

Calories

Calories come primarily from protein and fats. Calories control our cholesterol and glucose levels and convert to both energy and fat. When we increase our energy (calorie) intake and use less energy or lack activity in our daily life the fat in our body increases. Over time, this contributes to obesity. A sound diet should include fruits, whole grains, and vegetables, which are low in calories but include necessary fiber. (We should consume 25g of fiber every day.) Fifty to seventy percent of our calorie intake should also consist of carbohydrates.

Fats

While an excess of saturated fats is unhealthy, we do need some fats to fuel our bodies. Fats increase our cholesterol and while there are healthy fats (mono-unsaturated fats and poly-unsaturated fats) and unhealthy fats (saturated fats and trans-fats), there is also good cholesterol and bad cholesterol.

Trans and saturated fatty acids increase the bad cholesterol level (LDL—Low-Density Lipoprotein). These fats contribute to heart disease by building blockage later in arteries. Studies show that meals with high saturated fat and high trans-fat result in constricted blood vessels, making the blood more prone to clotting. For this reason, saturated fats should be limited to 10% of our total calorie consumption while trans-fat should be avoided. A small amount of saturated fat is essential for our body since it provides amino acids that control inflammation, generate new cells, and help the development of the brain.

Mono-unsaturated fats decrease the risk of heart disease by reducing the triglyceride cholesterol level, helping decrease joint inflammation, and reducing blood clotting in our bodies. Mono-unsaturated fats are found in canola oil, olive oil, peanut oil, and fish oils. Nuts are also a rich source of unsaturated fats. Poly-unsaturated fats, another fatty acid, make cell membranes and hormones for the body. Poly-unsaturated fats are available in vegetables oils like canola, corn, and safflower oils, as well as in seafood.

For good health, these three elements—sodium, calories, and fats— need to be monitored and adjusted regularly. Excess amounts can lead to obesity, which causes a number of health problems and puts stress on bones and joints. Too little leads to a person being underweight and increases the chance of infection.

The Good and Bad of a Healthy Diet

Evaluate your diet. A body needs some calories—in the form of proteins, carbohydrates, and different fats, including ten percent of saturated fats needed for energy. However, the food you eat should provide almost all the nutrients and vitamins your body needs. Some nutrients provide energy and strengthen our natural defense system against infections. Others keep our lungs healthy and help us control our weight. We can improve our consumption of nutrients by consuming real food like fruits, vegetables, whole grain breads, and cereals. Depletion of nutrients can lead to a feeling of fatigue, decrease in performance, or depression and other serious health problems. Organize your eating habits and maintain a balanced intake of proteins, carbohydrates, and fats. As we age, our caloric intake decreases, but our need for proteins, vitamins, and minerals does not change. As a result, we often end up supplementing with vitamins.

Dietary supplements can be instrumental in helping our bodies achieve a proper nutrient balance. **Probiotics** are "good bacteria"—a supplement that can aid in digestion and the functioning of the intestines. A probiotic, such as bifidobacterium, should be rich in culture count with at least ten strains. Yogurt is one well-known probiotic, recommended to me by surgeon L.G. Yerbie, MD. Other probiotic supplements are available at a vitamin store. Avoid probiotics containing sugars and look for recent cultures. They will be more effective than those close to the ending date on their package.

To start your day with energy, a **fiber**-rich cereal is an ideal breakfast. Throughout the day, other great choices for replenishing nutrients include broccoli, cabbage, cauliflower, beans, green leafy vegetables, berries, oranges, melons, apples, pears, peaches, and nuts. A well-nourished body will fight infection. When enough external nutrients are not available, the body will create energy by using body sugars and fats. This energy is transmitted to your muscles via oxygen. Muscle fibers rely on the oxidation system to complete the energy cycle. A low intensity workout increases our activity and makes our oxidation more effective, which improves our mental focus.

Oils are found in many foods today. Like other fat sources, there are good oils and harmful oils. **Fish oils** reduce the risk of coronary heart disease, give us energy, and increase bone mass. Fish oils contain Omega-3 fatty acids and can be found in salmon, sardines, rainbow trout, and albacore tuna or mackerel herring. According to the American Heart Association (AHA), Omega-3 contains EPA (eicosapentaenoic acid) and DHA (docosahexaenoic acid) fatty acids that protect us against heart disease. Research was conducted on an Eskimo diet where Omega-3 was found. Results showed that EPA and DHA decreased the triglycerides that make LDL cholesterol in the arteries and increase blood pressure. Omega-3 unclogs the deposition along the walls of arteries, thereby lowering body blood pressure. Omega-3 is also recommended by some ophthalmologists as being good for eye health. The AHA recommends eating fish twice a week for those who are not allergic to fish. Check with your health care provider to find out if Omega-3 is suitable for you.

Hydrogenated oils and shortenings, on the other hand, should be avoided. Oils are solidified through a process that uses nickel and aluminum as catalysts. While most of the catalysts are removed after solidification, during the purification process, some traces of the catalysts are left behind in the shortenings. These traces are harmful to our health. Any trace of hydrogenated oil increases cholesterol levels in our bodies.

The melting point of hydrogenated shortening is higher than our body temperatures. Without melting, digestion of hydrogenated shortening becomes very difficult and catalyst traces left behind accumulate in the body. According to Dr. Buzz Hentz, a retired chemistry professor from North Carolina State University, after many years of consumption of hydrogenated shortening, the accumulated traces may increase the chances of disease, so precautionary measures are always in order. (While not yet proven or disproven by the American Medical Association, early data suggests that there may be a link between years of hydrogenated oil intake and Alzheimer's disease.) Check food labels to avoid hydrogenated shortening in your foods. Some well-known sources are Crisco and other shortenings that claim to "taste like butter."

One published article goes so far as to say that foods containing hydrogenated oils are "probably the most toxic foods that we buy in our grocery stores." We have become accustomed to buying shortening, Crisco, for example, to make cakes, bake cookies, or fry foods. Advertisements of hydrogenated oils that 'taste like butter' entice us into thinking that hydrogenated oil is as good as butter. Butter, however, has a melting temperature that matches the human body temperature; therefore, it is easier to digest. All varieties of hydrogenated oils are considered harmful to our body and should be avoided. As an alternative, use pure butter in limited quantities and reduce your overall intake of saturated fats.

Love   Live   Laugh

We will still be tempted to eat foods fried in shortening. To help digest such foods, I suggest that you drink some warm liquid with it. Consider hot tea (Chinese style), warm wine (Japanese style), or simply warm (not very hot) water. Ayurvedic principles recommend sipping lukewarm water throughout the day. Hot liquids are not recommended because they can irritate the esophagus. Europeans drink wine with cheese for the same effect as warm water. Such precautions will help clear the esophagus before condensation of the shortening. Condensation causes coughing. Warm liquids help to melt the shortening and aid digestion.

Whenever possible, avoid very cold water with your foods. The body should digest all the food that we consume before the oils get a chance to solidify in the arteries. Solidified foods are slow to digest and can upset the system.

As a rule, don't underestimate the importance of water. We should drink eight to twelve cups of water every day. A gastro internist advised me that drinking two glasses of water in the morning helps normalize stomach acidity, in addition to preventing dehydration. Here are some other important facts about water:

- A body can't function in a dehydrated state.
- Water replaces sweat and urine loss.
- Water distributes proteins, carbohydrates, and fat.
- Water distributes and controls sugars, curbs hunger, and increases energy.
- Recommend warm water in winter and ice-free water in summer.

Good sources of calcium include cereal; Lactaid, low-fat, or soy milk; ricotta, Swiss, mozzarella, or cheddar cheese; and orange juice. Calcium contributes to our bone mass, which can protect our hips and lumbar vertebrae from fractures.

Love   Live   Laugh

Some foods, including pineapple, ginger, berries, and green vegetables, are known to reduce arthritic pains. The Human Nutrition Research Center at Tufts University wrote that compounds in blueberries mitigate inflammation and oxidation damage, which is associated with aging and deficits in our memory motor functions. Eating pineapple is very highly recommended in different literatures.

Cured meats are foods to avoid. Cured meats contain nitrites. Nitrites are found in cold cuts, refined grains, red meats, and French fries. These items are linked to high cholesterol levels and may cause inflammation or increase stress in the lungs. Harvard University defined processed meats as meats that are preserved by smoking, curing, salting, or with the addition of chemical preservatives. Their study found that such processed meats contribute to a 42% higher risk of heart disease and a 19% higher risk of diabetes.

Red wine is advertised as good for the heart in that it contains a small amount of resveratrol compound that may contribute to slowing down the aging process. My own research finds that red wine does not contain enough resveratrol compounds to meet these needs. For overall good health and weight management, recent literature suggests that reducing alcohol consumption and avoiding smoking helps.

While it is difficult to cut down on foods that you love to eat, or that are tempting for their taste, try spoon-sized helpings. This practice should become part of your ongoing diet management.

Weight Loss

The formula for weight loss is a simple one. ***Expend more calories than you take in.*** However, while calorie management is critical, it is important to note that genealogy, age, sex, race, and our height play a role in weight management and our tendency toward being heavy or lean. Managing weight and diet must be considered in the same realm. A Stanford

Love   Live   Laugh

University study states that if you are worried about your weight, a simple DNA test can predict what kind of diet will work for you – either a low-carbohydrate or a low-fat diet. For weight management over the long term, consider genealogy before targeting a specific weight for your body.

In one weight-loss study, a group was divided into three different genotypes: low-carbohydrate-diet responders, low-fat-diet responders, and balanced-diet responders. Researchers found that when a proper diet was followed, a person could lose two to three times more weight over a one-year period of time, compared to an insufficient diet plan. Food not only gives us nourishment and fulfills our body's needs; it also delights our taste buds, bringing enjoyment to eating. Diet management and any diet plan should consider this balance.

Successful diet management does not imply that you should forget the foods that you enjoy, rather the quantity and the frequency with which you indulge. The motivation and control to manage your food intake lies within you. You may decide to splurge once a week on the foods that you have not eaten recently while for the other six days you limit yourself to healthy choices. Splurging once in a while reduces your temptation to eat certain foods. You will find that over time your appetite for certain foods will change. As you achieve your weight loss or weight management goals, you will gain momentum and enthusiasm to eat and enjoy healthy foods.

TV advertisements generally lead us to believe that losing weight is a quick and simple task. In fact, dieting for a short period of time often backfires. Many people gain weight after the dieting period is done. A relatively gradual loss of weight due to sensible diet management and activity provides us long-term health benefits while maintaining weight at a desired level.

Your exercises may include walking, hiking, jogging, stair climbing, dancing, playing tennis, or exercising in a gym. All these activities help reduce fats by burning extra calories during diet management. See more on

Love   Live   Laugh

these activities and exercises in Chapter: 'Stretching and Walking for Health'. Like your weight management plan, your exercise program should be designed with respect to your genealogy and your objectives. Healthy changes in your body will be seen gradually over time. Do not expect them overnight. Remember that your genealogy is different from others; therefore, do not compare your appearance with others. *Beauty is in the eye of the beholder.*

Here are some tips for effective weight loss:

- Eat small meals at regular intervals and avoid stuffing yourself.
- Post reminders that may motivate, engage, and lead you to healthy choices.
- Keep healthy snacks on hand for occasional treats.
- Start each day with a healthy breakfast.
- Eat fruits and vegetables every day.
- Incorporate yogurt into your diet to maintain good functionality of intestines.
- Stay active. Exercise and stretch regularly.
- Quit smoking.

Statistics

- Someone suffers a stroke every 45 seconds. You can prevent such occurrences. Help change the statistics by paying more attention to your diet. Learn from the healthy habits of other cultures. You can cut the risk of having a stroke by 50% when you are active for at least thirty minutes a day, eat five daily servings of fruits and vegetables, and avoid cigarettes and excess alcohol.

Love   Live   Laugh

- A study published in the Archives of Internal Medicine involving more than 5,000 women related that the vitamin B (including B-6 and B-12) reduced the risk of macular degeneration in women.

- A joint study by an Australian and a Vietnamese, regarding a link between bone density and the diet habits of more than 2,700 people, was published in the American Journal of Clinical Nutrition by Tuan Nguyen. The study explained that vegetarians had five percent less bone density compared to non-vegetarians. Bone density among people who ate meat compared to those who ate eggs and dairy products (excluding meat and seafood) was practically similar.

- Another study involving half a million older men and women found that calcium products protected them against cancer. Foods with high calcium were more effective in absorption of calcium compared to the available calcium supplements. When calcium supplements are used, avoid consuming more than 600mg of calcium at one time.

- A study found that daily vitamins and balanced calcium (possibly calcium coming from milk products) cuts the risk of older adults falling down or breaking bones, especially hipbones.

- Metabolic syndrome that causes the potential for heart disease, stroke, and diabetes results from a cluster of risk factors, for example, elevated triglycerides, increased blood pressure and blood sugar, and low levels of HDL cholesterol, or abdominal fats. Ask your physician to specify healthy levels by which you can measure those requisite levels.

- A study of 20,000 British men and women published in British Medical Journal showed that the incidence of obesity and chronic disease skyrocketed, especially after retirement.

.

Love   Live   Laugh

- A publication in *U.S. News & World Report* written by Deborah Kotz indicated that a lack of exercise or physical activity does not fully compensate for the intake of excess calories or over-eating. The result is obesity. The World Health Organization (WHO), at the European Association for the Study of Obesity conference, estimated in 2005 that about 1.6 million adults were overweight. WHO also estimated that at least 400 million are obese.

If you are struggling with obesity, find the root cause of your problem rather than using excuses and blaming others or food itself. Shoulder your responsibility since only your sincere efforts will give you the self-control you need in order to reach a healthy goal. Self-help is a substitute for well-intended professional help. Your success depends upon you and your will. Manage your diet and physical activities.

Jim, at the gym I go to, had been exercising over two years to manage his obese condition. He was not successful since he ignored to manage his diet. In last 3 months, he decided to manage his diet in addition to his exercise plan. He lost 25 pounds in this period and his body is shaping up. His blood pressure is now normal. This example shows that you need to manage both your diet and the exercises.

An article in *Investment Business Daily* on August 31, 2009 discussed the importance of preventing obesity. The study, conducted by scientists at UCLA and the University of Pittsburg, involved elderly people. The scientists concluded that the brains of obese people degenerate and have 8% less brain tissue than an average-weight person. Someone who is merely overweight has 4% less brain tissue. Furthermore, the brains of the obese sampling looked 16 years older than the brains of the normal-weight sampling. This study was the first time that personal weight and brain degeneration were linked.

Organic Foods

To sum up, protein is essential for the maintenance of muscles. A small amount of saturated fats (10%) supply all the amino acids that a body needs. Both protein and saturated fats exist in meats and eggs, butter, cheese, milk, coconut, and palm oils. Saturated fats can raise blood cholesterol in a body. Eating bacon, salami, sausage, hot-dogs and other processed meats can raise the risk of heart disease and diabetes. A body needs cholesterol for normal body functions; however, the body itself makes more than enough cholesterol for its needs. Attention should be given to foods that may absorb pesticides. Brierly Wright, M.S., a registered dietician, suggests we consider eating the following foods in their organic states, while buying other organic foods may not be necessary:

Apple	Strawberries	Celery
Nectarines	Cherries	Kale
Grapes	Peaches	Bell Peppers
Pears	Lettuce	Carrots

Recent yahoo internet printed the healthiest meals by Leatherhead, food research, England.

- Salmon terrine, mixed leaf salad with virgin olive oil dressing, chicken casserole with lentils and mixed vegetables and high-fiber multigrain roll.
- Dessert – Yogurt-base topped with walnuts and sugar-free caramel sauce. This desert is good for digestion, blood glucose control, and teeth.
- Snacks – Walnuts and sugar-free spearmint chewing gum with xylitol.

Love   Live   Laugh

If your system get upset because of stool constrain, solve it by drinking 2-4 fl. oz. of natural Prune juice.

Above aspects will manage your health. The management and improvement of your health is extremely important and you are the controller. Consider above information will help your health.

Most film actresses manage their diets for six days in a week and splurge once a week. **You can do it too**.

Chapter 4

Brain & Memory Stimulation

Shan, a student in my class, and many others tell me that they keep forgetting things. What can they do to improve their brain power and increase their memory?

In my opinion, you need to understand the functioning of your brain and all the activities it does. You may choose to do some brain exercises by solving different types of problems that will strengthen your brain cells and increase the neuron count. The brain is a mystery. To improve your memory you need to work on your brain cells so that the neuron count stops shrinking. This can be accomplished by keeping your brain active.

The brain is a miracle, even for scientists. Nerve cell production in the human brain is directly related to our learning and our memory, according to a study from the University of Florida. Our body senses gather information and position the brain as the controller of all planning, decision making, and related actions. Scientists are still struggling to determine what exactly stimulates the nerve cell production.

Today's technology considers the brain to be a body's computer. In reality, the brain is more powerful than any existing electronic computer. Computers need electrical impulses for its operation; so does the brain. These are developed from your body juices that are nurtured to transmit information to different parts of your body. Body juices are created from your positive thoughts. Positive thinking, your senses, and actions become an essential part of your brain functionality and its stimulation.

You can improve your memory by using a few memory-building exercises. These exercises include keeping your brain cells healthy. Keep your brain cells healthy by engaging yourself in activities like reading,

Love   Live   Laugh

solving crossword puzzles, visiting museums, solving some complex problems (like Sudoku), or enjoying a card game on a regular basis.

A state of happiness helps maintain mental health, along with your senses of smell, touch, taste, hearing, and sight. Writing also contributes to good mental health. As you maximize your involved senses, you will see that your memory of your actions and thoughts increases. To avoid forgetting, you may repeat the same information many times in your head. Such consistent repeating in your mind will increase your mental stress. I believe that such mental stress can be reduced if you write that information on a piece of paper. It will relieve your mental stress and you will not forget your thought.

How are your senses and your experiences related to your memorization? The information that you sense or gather is processed by your brain to help increase your focus. A higher level of focus increases your memory by strengthening your brain.

In addition to these factors, a good rest or a good night's sleep relieves mental strain (stress). A balanced diet that includes vitamins, supplements, and especially Omega-3 keeps the brain in a healthy condition.

As a part of your fitness program, you need to keep your brain in a healthy state. When the brain and its nervous system are programmed appropriately, the brain will operate at an optimum healthy level. Researchers have confirmed that after a certain age the brain cells, or brain neurons, start to shrink. Neurons do not die off, however, as long as your brain stays active by doing some sort of activity. In fact, brain cells actually strengthen the network of neurons in your brain.

All kinds of activities build your agility and resistance to diseases. Happy people are likely to maintain their mental health by keeping their brains active. Also, physical and mental exercises with a positive attitude will enhance or maintain your memory. A smile on your face, positive thoughts, and a few physical exercises help pass impulses from your brain to all parts of your body.

A French study says that the human brain is capable of multi-tasking depending upon your incentive and your priorities. The front lobe of the brain divides itself to accomplish different tasks at the same time.

Cardiovascular exercises pump oxygenated blood to the body. The brain receives a high percentage of the oxygenated blood, which creates new neurons and new brain cells. This scenario will keep you alert, happy, and healthy. Design a few physical exercises for yourself; exercises that suit your body. Plan how often you will do these exercises over a week-long period. Include cardiovascular exercise as part of this program.

I explained to my student, Shan, that we do lose instant memory with age. However, when we work hard to recollect our thoughts, the memory will return. We can alleviate memory loss by regenerating new brain cells and nerves. This is managed by a network of neurons.

Since the brain controls all the bodily functions, including our memory and our thinking power, it becomes essential for us to maintain our brain by following the characteristics of our active brain:

- Stay flexible in your thinking. Do not allow excuses or negativity to misalign your thought process. Excuses are harmful to the soul.

- Excuses and procrastination are poisonous to your thoughts. These are meant to let you escape from your responsibilities.

- Always think positively to enhance your mood and enjoyment.

- Develop your thoughts to believe in love by allowing yourself to love life, nature, beauty, and your surroundings. Divine power will gather within you to make you happy.

- Increase your love for others and in return others will love you. In addition, your actions will bring appreciation from others for you.

- Allow yourself to unfold naturally to allow your blood and adrenaline to circulate in your body for your health.

- Do not complain. It is an insult to your surroundings. Complaints will reduce your enjoyment in life.

- Allow yourself time to relax and enjoy everything under the sun.

- Be creative and free to attain the great gift of your imagination and self-esteem.

- Develop faith in yourself and get rid of fears. Faith helps and allows you to master and resolve difficult tasks and situations.

- Play a musical instrument that you enjoy. I understand that piano is the most desirable musical instrument for exercising your brain since it involves thinking of the musical notes, and movement of your fingers and feet in unison. Our brain controls all these actions.

- Visit interesting places that you may have dreamed of. Add to your enjoyment by asking friends to accompany you. You can socialize and laugh with them during your trip.

> *Where there is love there is life.* Mahatma Gandhi

You may have heard the slogan: "The mind is a terrible thing to waste." What good is a great body if you lose your mental capacity?

This slogan is a reminder that you need to do something to maintain, develop, and sharpen your brain. The brain has the unimaginable power of thinking, planning, and resolving difficult tasks.

Love   Live   Laugh

The brain never rests since it stays active even when we are resting or sleeping. The brain works and gains knowledge to bring different outcomes. It searches different circumstances that will help it to cope with new ideas and situations. It will align itself with the present and the future so it can make changes. Mental power can change human behavior and lifestyle. Focus on what you can do rather than what you can't do.

Your positive focus will be on what you can accomplish rather than what you can't.

Develop different ways for your senses to help you become a problem solver and a thinker. The solutions to problems will entice you to be happy and will bring you a sense of accomplishment and self-confidence.

The brain can process information faster than any electronic equipment. The brain gathers information from the senses and all sensed information is passed to the brain cells. Depending upon the nature of the information, the brain will affect a person's moods and reactions. The brain, being so active, continuously produces vital messages coded into electrical impulses that are transmitted to the elements of the human body to conduct the body's functions.

After retirement, try not to miss the job where you may have spent forty or more years of your life. During this period, you may have missed the ambitious project that you always wanted to do. After retirement, I suggest that you plan your future life and consider what you missed that you now want to accomplish. Your desires should bring happiness and energy. I am not saying that you should not appreciate your achievements during your working life. But do look toward your new future plans. Such planning will lead you toward a stress-free, enjoyable, happy, and rewarding life in the future. What can be more rewarding?

All this planning and mental exercise helps in slowing down the aging process. You will develop your memory so it becomes sharp. A University of Florida study states, "If we can increase the regeneration of nerve cells, we can alleviate or prevent memory loss in humans."

The important thing to remember is that you should never give up because of your age. Continue planning and thinking like a young adult. Eat a balanced diet of the right foods containing vitamins and calcium for your body's needs. Keep your mental stress at bay and have a good night sleep. Increase your concentrated focus.

At the age of 75, I decided to change my field of interest after my retirement. I play bridge and go to the gym for my fitness exercises. I teach others the game of bridge, breathing and meditation techniques, and healthy living. I took a personal training course to learn how muscular functions relate to different physical exercises, and how to administer CPR/AED. I help others stay healthy and keep mental alertness at all times. I feel young all the time!

Alertness and happiness are the positive nodes that will create new nerve cells, energy cells, and neurons in the brain to control the aging process, thus helping us to retain our memory. Psychologically, we all need a social circle to support us and to help fulfill our emotional needs. It provides assurance to know that someone cares. Socialization is the best way to accomplish this.

Effective points:

- Write down your thoughts and manage your schedule. This will help you to organize your ideas and your plans.
- Increase your memorization by writing and mentally repeating. Help maintain your memory for the long haul.
- Develop your methodology and pay attention to completing your tasks.
- Add new information to your existing knowledge.

Love   Live   Laugh

Surveys indicate that the world will spend 604 billion dollars in 2010 to help Alzheimer's sufferers. This cost is expected to rise by 83% by the year 2030. Avoid being part of this group by helping yourself with mental exercises and precautions.

Here is some information regarding our brain.

The left eye information is processed by the right side of the brain and vice versa. Similarly, the left side of brain handles the right side body functions and information. The frontal lobe of the brain handles planning, emotions, and control capabilities. The functions of both sides of the brain are described below:

Left side Brain senses	Right side Brain senses
Logical Sequential	Random
Rational	Intuitive
Analytical	Holistic Synthesizer
Objective	Subjective
Analyze information by parts	Visualize as a whole
Scholastic and Accuracy	Focus on Aesthetic, Feeling & Creativity

The brain weighs only 3 pounds and has 100 billion cells. Cells are also called neurons. Neurons communicate with the body by using different chemicals (called transmitters). Information transmits from one neuron to the next. All body communication occurs through the spinal cord while hearings and sights have direct access to the brain. The brain consumes 40-50% of a body's oxidized blood.

Love   Live   Laugh

Good and bad decisions affect the present and the future. For example, every action or decision of our elders affects the coming generations. The coming generation ends up paying for their decisions. Practically, it is very important to consider all the facts and aspects with our sharp minds before making any decisions. Develop the habit of analyzing many different possibilities before accepting them with known implications.

Help not to lose your memory due to age by keeping yourself alert.

Recently, a nutrition journal published an article about the benefits of Omega-3, the unsaturated fatty acids found in fish. It helps seniors' thinking ability. A test was conducted involving people in the age group of 75 to 85 years old. (Refer to information on Omega-3 in Chapter: 'Healthy Foods & Diet Management' and in a nutritional journal.) Omega-3's benefits were the result of a study of the diet of Eskimos. The American Health Association (AHA) accepts these benefits.

A woman who feels enervated or who is losing her memory after menopause may consider modifying her diet by including vitamin B, Omega-3, calcium, and other food nutrients recommended by her physician or her dietician. Literature suggests that calcium and bone density will help her maintain her memory.

Managing your diet and doing mental and physical exercises will help boost your cognitive aging functions. Published data on May 11, 2009 in the *Proceedings of the National Academy of Sciences* journal suggests that daydreaming is an important cognitive state where you will unconsciously exercise your brain by turning your attention from an immediate task to sorting through problems in your life.

A surprising experiment regarding brain activity during daydreaming was conducted by Christoff who used MRI tests to view results at the University of British Columbia in Canada. He concluded, "Our brains are very active when we daydream – much more active than when we focus on routine tasks." The study also showed that the brain's 'executive network,' associated with high level, complex problem solving, was lit up during the daydreaming tests.

Intelligent Quotient (IQ) is defined as 'the intelligence that has the ability to learn, understand or deal with new or trying situations with logical and reasoning skills.' These skills change with age depending upon your experience and exposure to various situations. A person with a high IQ becomes successful only when effort is applied with self-confidence and self-assurance. Effort is required with our ability to accomplish or complete any task.

Develop an infinite faith in yourself with passion, energy, wisdom, and knowledge.

Chapter 5

Toning your Muscles

Our activities and exercises tone our muscles. Activities involve walking, running, yoga exercises or fitness exercising, breathing and meditation. Such activities not only strengthen our muscles, they make our body f

lexible and stress-free.

Yoga is not just about relaxation and meditation; it is a 5,000-year-old exercise. This type of exercise will help to reduce anxiety, improve muscle strength and flexibility, and tone your muscles and blood circulation. Consistent yoga exercises will help both the toning of muscles and relaxation.

Stretching exercises lubricate the joints and muscles that go through a complete range of motions flexing bone mass, physically strengthening tendons, ligaments, body muscles and lumbar muscles. Stretching is important for toning the body.

Our blood pressure is generally lower in the morning and the evening. It starts going up as the day progresses, and reaches its maximum reading close to noontime. As we wake up, our bodies start secreting adrenaline and hormones that increase demand of more oxygen by our bodies. Stretching for 15 minutes to fulfill this bodily need helps our system get normalized.

Shan, stretches are essential for your muscles and body to get on an energetic path and to enhance your mood. The stretches don't have to be vigorous. The objective is to gain some energy in the body, feel healthy, and acquire mental alertness. It starts the day a lot more efficiently and effectively.

Love   Live   Laugh

While lying in bed, start stretching the muscles in your toes, feet, ankles and legs. Toeing and stretching your feet inward, outward, and rotating them in both directions will help your tendons, leg muscles, and the upper part of your thighs. Each stretch may be held for a count of 5. Repeat all the stretches in different directions before sitting up in your bed. Before getting out of bed, take a few deep breaths to provide oxygen to your body. This practice will massage your legs and thighs.

After your inhalations, stretch your neck, arms, fingers, and hands behind your back and above your head a few times. Exercise your eyes by blinking them as you get out of bed. Stand in an optimal posture—tall and high—with your shoulders even, and stretch your arms horizontally, out to both sides, at shoulder level. Twist your oblique in a circular motion as you move your arms. Do this twice. Look to each side, at shoulder level, and when you do, turn your head to look as far behind you as possible. Do this twice. These exercises will stretch your neck muscles.

Stand with your head upright and backbone (spine) vertical, feeling tall and high. Raise both arms up by your sides and as you do, inhale and pull your bellybutton inward. Exhale as you bring your arms down. During each breathing sequence, you may lift your steps up and down like a march. Do laughing yoga five times. This means laugh loudly as you raise your arms parallel above your head.

Stand with your feet apart. Raise your arms out to your sides at shoulder level. To set up the triangle pose, twist your upper body to one side, bending to lower one hand down while raising the other hand as high as possible. Do this two to three times on each side.

Add a few squats to your morning routine by standing with your back near a wall and your feet separated to your body width. Bend your knees and sink slowly to a chair position. Hold your hands in front of you and count to 5. Return to a standing position and repeat the sequence three to five times.

Love   Live   Laugh

Stand in a warrior pose. Start with a triangle pose and turn your right foot 90 degrees. Bend your right knee above your right foot. With arms kept at shoulder level, turn your head to your right above your shoulder, looking at the wall on your right. Now, bend your upper body to your right and place your elbow over your right thigh. Raise your left hand high above your head. Hold to a count of five. Repeat the warrior pose to your left side.

Triangle pose, warrior pose and laughing exercises are yoga exercises. These will massage your lymph system gently and apply a small amount of pressure to your muscles. Consistent massages and movements will energize your body for your daily chores. Hold something stationary if you need some support to keep your balance whenever you may need it. You may relax your muscles with warm water. Warming the muscles make them feel good.

Be sure to drink water during the day and keep your body normalized.

"Stay healthy with a positive outlook and eating balanced diet."

Chapter 6

Stretching & Walking for Health

You need to develop a habit of doing a few stretches in the morning and going for a morning walk. After you wake up in the morning, a 20-30 minute walk is healthy for you. Stretching exercises will help keep your body flexibility for the whole day; your bones will get healthier and stronger and your cardiovascular breathing will improve for your physical health.

Walking is the easiest cardiovascular exercise that you can do to enhance your heart rate and health. Walking is the simplest means to manage your metabolism. Walking burns calories, controls blood pressure, manages blood sugar and diabetes, and reduces heart disease. In addition to this list, walking helps your knees and legs, and the muscles and tendons surrounding them.

In my Breathing and Meditation class, a woman told me that she used to breathe uncomfortably during and after her walks. The breathing techniques in this book (refer to Chapter: 'Breathing Techniques') controlled her breathing to a comfortable level. She stopped feeling uncomfortable during her walks.

An optimal body posture—tall and high—is essential during all stretches and exercises. During walks, develop this posture by paying attention to your posture all the times. Look straight in front of you, not at the ground, during your walks.

If you look down to the ground, your neck is bent and you may end up bending your spine. Under this type of strain, you may easily lose control of keeping your optimal posture. Optimal posture will allow you to inhale more oxygen to enhance the health of your lymph system with the proper circulation of oxidized blood.

Love   Live   Laugh

Inhale and exhale a few deep breaths before starting your morning walk. It will reduce your fatigue. It will expand your lungs and will help your walk. It will increase your heart rate. Your lung expansion increases your ability to circulate more oxygenated blood throughout your body dispensing carbon dioxide and other toxins. It will make you feel energetic throughout your day.

If you are not in the habit of morning walks or doing exercises, you should start this practice slowly. You may initially walk short distances and for short periods. Develop enjoyment of your walks. If walking outside is a problem, walk inside your home. Keep your walk periods within your comfort zone. As your muscles get used to your walks, the time, distance, and speed of your walking will improve.

Control your walking speed so as not to gasp or feel short of breath. If your breathing becomes difficult just relax by taking some deep breaths. To avoid gasping during your walk, I recommend that before your walk, you practice some breathing exercises as I have described in this book. It will help you with breathing problems, and will allow you to enjoy your walks.

With a consistent habit of morning walking, you may increase your walking capacity and attain some speed. A brisk walk increases the heart rate for a good cardiovascular exercise. Consider your breathing capacity as you increase speed. Breathing fresh air and seeing colorful birds during your walk will be enjoyable for you.

As you raise your heart rate, you are exercising your heart muscles and burning a higher number of calories. Brisk walks significantly increase the endurance level and maintain the health of the heart. This kind of healthy living reduces the risk of developing macular degeneration – a leading cause of vision loss.

Enjoyment is the key to staying motivated with your walking program. Add enjoyment to your walks. Morning weather is congenial for healthy walking. Increase enjoyment of morning exercise by watching and

Love   Live   Laugh

enjoying the natural sceneries surrounding you. You may walk in the company of your friends. If you prefer, listen to some music during your walks. Flexing muscles, enjoying the environment, and feeling relaxed are the optimal aims of morning walks.

Ordinarily our bodies do not get dehydrated even during a one-hour walk, but you must be very careful and keep some liquid with you. You may take a few sips of water or liquid as you walk for longer periods. In a humid environment, you may sweat a lot and reduce your body fluids. Pay attention to your thirst. Feeling thirsty is a precursor of dehydration. Drink some liquid (or water) slowly to quench your thirst. Rest helps your heart rate return to normal. After feeling normal, you may drink as much liquid as you like. Please, do not gulp liquid quickly when your heart is beating fast. Gulping liquids at this state can make the liquid flow in the wrong part of your body. Slowly sip liquid to restore body energy.

Walking under a hot sun may not only dehydrate you, it can also give you heat stroke. In a dehydrated condition, it is generally recommended that you drink 10 ounces of non-carbonated liquid(s) containing glucose every 20-30 minutes.

Cardiovascular walks, and reducing your stress, contribute to healthy living. Stress can be reduced by proper rest, and managing your diet and work habits, among other things. Meditation is a perfect solution for reducing your stress. Here are a few points for your healthy living:

- Structure an exercise plan that you can easily follow.
- Maintain your sleeping and resting habits by keeping a schedule.
- Reduce your mental anxiety level by talking about your problems. It is good therapy.
- Manage your dietary habits. Digest food that is well balanced.
- Set realistic goals for your life.

For a long and a healthy life, you must do stretches regularly and go for walks. Moderate and enjoyable activities should be included. Walking in the morning is a great cardiovascular exercise. For strengthening particular body muscles, your exercise program should include that body muscle. Tone the lower body, upper body, and abdominal muscles, in addition to improving your posture, reducing body fat, and increasing cardio functions to lead a healthy life.

"A healthy life slows down the aging process."

Chapter 7

Resting & Being Stress-free

We all have certain conditions that trigger stress. Our reaction to these triggers determines how that stress affects us. First, let's define stress using a concrete example.

If you hold something in front of you for a moment, you are very comfortable. You don't feel pain holding it. When you hold the same item for a longer period, you start feeling some strain in your arm or shoulder. When you hold the same item for a whole day, you will feel a great deal of strain in your body. You become quite uncomfortable. Holding the same item created different stress levels.

Stress appears when you are required to perform certain tasks consistently over a long period. To reduce your stress level, as you may have concluded from the above example, break long periods of time into shorter periods. Stress management implies that you plan rest breaks whenever you are carrying a heavy load. This will help you manage your stress level efficiently.

Stress can come from many different sources. It may come from sadness. Sadness upsets your system and makes you feel dejected. Even when you are trying not to get stressed, many circumstances may lead you to feel stress in your life.

Here's an example: You have an interview and on the way your car gives up. You get stressed. Another example: You are selected as the best pitcher on your team, but while practicing, a nerve in your hand starts acting up. You get stressed. In both examples, you had an opportunity but circumstances put you behind.

Love   Live   Laugh

Stress is common among us. We need to learn how to deal with our stress and manage it within our control. Your improved situation will improve your decision-making, help you deal with anger or grief, and enhance your ability to communicate with others.

Worry and nervousness cause stress and release toxins into the body. This situation will increase blood pressure and heart rate, and the body will release adrenaline cortical and other hormones and chemicals. Stress interferes with the immune system and will increase cholesterol levels and reduce breathing capacity. When stress is unmanaged, it may cause headaches, digestive troubles, and sleep problems.

Certain diseases and illnesses are associated with the emotions. Mental stress causes carotid artery dilation that increases the blood pressure causing heart rate to go higher. Such physical disorders may make a person act irritably and irresponsibly.

It is important to learn some healthy ways to release stress and attain peace in your mind. Some stress management involves exercises like Yoga, stretches, meditation, and deep breathing. Before you go to work on Monday morning, some relaxation and a good night's sleep will help you reduce your strain, otherwise your body may feel fatigued - upsetting your natural rhythms.

Tai Chi exercises help seniors make a few physical movements to reduce your arthritic problems and improve their physical balance. Many use Tai Chi not only to promote relaxation but also to develop their mood and body balance. The happiness that comes from good moods leads you to positivity and your well-being. Your positive attitude will bring additional happiness. Avoid negative environments and reduce your stress and anxiety. Stay happy by enhancing your self-esteem.

To maintain your mental and physical condition, relax your body. That includes increasing your breathing capacity. Resting, engaging in recreational activities, and getting plenty of sleep are vital for good health.

Love   Live   Laugh

When you meet your friends and family, laugh with them. Under depressed or tired conditions, resting can become a lifesaver that rejuvenates the body cells.

Mentally remembering a solution to a problem may not be easy, I suggest that you write down the solution to alleviate your mental stress. Revisit the written solution to evaluate before implementing it. Your faith in the development of a solution will relax you. You may take a deep breath of relief. The results will help you regain your strength and vitality, your self-faith and your energy while reducing your stress. Rest and relaxation reduces the discomfort, headaches, and anxiety increasing your memory, and normalizing the blood pressure.

A relaxed brain develops new ideas and your concentration helps to develop a few solutions. Your strength and your consistent attempts will lead you to an appropriate solution.

Psychologists believe that getting away from stressful environments reduces stress levels. This will be healthier and more effective for you. In general, it is necessary to resolve the issue that is causing stress in you.

- Identify the cause of your stress—the cause is a stressor. Look for the obvious causes of stressors. It may include a change in your lifestyle or a family problem.

- Once you determine the stressor, engage in positive thinking to determine the best resolution for the stressor.

- If your mind does not stay positive over a long period, try to practice by staying positive for 15 minutes at a stretch and get used to the positive patterns.

- Incrementally increase your positivity period beyond 15 minutes to encompass the majority of your day. You've developed yourself to be a positive thinker.

Love   Live   Laugh

- Practice relaxing your body and mind with your eyes closed. Take deep breaths and concentrate on every part of your body in a meditating mode and eliminate stressful thoughts by getting away from your hectic and stressful life.

- Increase your consciousness to reasons, apathy, pride, courage, and your willingness to look ahead with neutrality to implement your ideas. When you uplift your vision, your spirit and pride feel good and you will get peace and love.

- To relax yourself, listen to music or do projects that interest you. Create your own music by helping people and your associates.

- Whenever you are feeling stressed, close your eyes, inhale deeply and exhale slowly to calm your nerves. Concentrate on your breathing and not on your problems.

- You may perform a few stretch exercises to circulate your blood. This helps to loosen muscule tension.

- Communicate your problems to close friends in whom you can confide. This will help reduce your stress. We are social creatures and a social network is essential for us.

When you feel tired or stressed, take a "**power-nap**." A power-nap is sleeping for a period of 20 to 30 minutes. It is a great way to relax. A power-nap will revitalize your energy and eliminate your stress. It refreshes and energizes your senses to help you increase your productivity and your decision-making capability. Practice helps develop these improvements.

It is important that your power-nap be limited to a short period and no more than an hour. The drawback of a longer nap is that it puts you in a deeper sleep phenomenon (REM) that will make you feel lethargic or may give you a slight headache. Short power-naps tend to not produce these side effects.

Love   Live   Laugh

Although there is no conclusive proof that ulcers and other diseases develop with stress, many medical journals indicate that they are the side effects of stress. Medical science recommends meditation for rest and relaxation. Reduce your cholesterol by decreasing your LDL (a bad cholesterol level) and improving your HDL (a good cholesterol level).

Barbara Stillwell, a UNC director for Nursing Practitioners at the medical school, mentioned on a program on National Public Radio program that emotional and stress psychology can cause different medical symptoms where medical test results can't relate to the cause. The patient may need an opportunity to talk about his/her problem rather than taking medication. She gave an example of a patient in England who developed a swallowing problem after the death of her husband. It turned out that she was suffering from a traumatic experience. She needed to express her feelings. All of her test related to swallowing problems were negative.

I suggest that before you seek medical help, go through the stress relieving points I provide. Look at your list of traumatic experiences and try to pinpoint, if possible, the possible cause(s) of your stress. The steps or techniques I mentioned may improve your condition. If your condition does not improve, seek professional help.

A report of the National Heart, Lung, and Blood Institute indicates that the average American's blood pressure is rising. More people are becoming obese. Only 41% of Americans have normal blood pressure. High blood pressure is a silent killer due to strokes, heart attacks, or kidney failure. Blood pressure may not be easy to manage simply through diet. Resting and stress reduction are the natural means that play a very important part in our lives to manage our blood pressure and our health.

Chapter 8

Success Stories of Diet Management & Exercises

Losing weight is a healthy step to managing metabolic syndrome and feeling better. Planning and sticking with managed eating habits help us to maintain our desired weight. Here I have included examples of people who exercised regularly, managed their diet to a small degree, and lost between 27 and 30 pounds. Exercising and the management of diet does help us to stay healthy.

Mr. Arthur Wyche – I met Arthur at my health club. He manages his exercise program with the help of an advisor. He used an elliptical cardio-machine for one hour, 5 days a week. He used minimum weights to stretch his muscles. He told me that he had always been a small eater and did not need to change his eating habits except to manage his intake of beer.

By following his exercise program and reducing his beer consumption, he lost 27 pounds over 8 months. He now looks and feels very healthy at the age of 55. He was not initially convinced that he would lose any weight; however, he decided to follow the exercise program since he had nothing to lose except the weight.

Mr. Mo Asad – When I met Mo, he had lot of weight to lose. He went on a crash program where he managed his diet, especially his rice intake. He exercised a lot. He exercised 5 times a week with heavy weights. Eventually, he added cardiovascular workouts to his exercise program. All his efforts paid off and he lost 30 pounds within 3 months.

Love   Live   Laugh

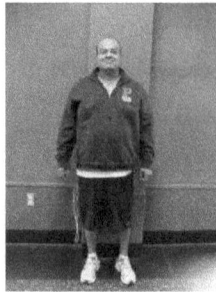

Lucy Danziger writes on the Internet about Jullian Michaels, that in her jam-packed schedule, she prioritizes her workout and her eating habits. Jullian would like to feel potent, capable, confident, and strong. To her, exercise is about building her body and managing her strength.

Looking at these examples, including the example of Jim in Chapter: 'Healthy Foods and Diet Management', and evaluating their feelings, I reiterate that exercising and diet management help to lose and manage your weight. It gives strength without the need of any kind of medicine. Muscle building may be a slow process but if you dedicate yourself to such a commitment, you will achieve favorable results for your health, including a reduction of your medical expenses.

LOSE WEIGHT - LIVE BETTER

Section 2: Body Physiology and Stretch Exercises

Scope of Section 2

This section will provide you with an understanding of your body's muscles and ligaments. This information is very valuable because it will help you understand what different stretches your body can handle, and what effects the stretches will have on increasing your endurance and stability. The stretches and muscular exercises will keep all parts of your body flexible, functional, and healthy. In addition, it will improve your body's immune system.

Before starting an exercise routine you must warm-up your body. The warm-ups will keep your body energetic as your cardio-respiratory system and blood starts to circulate. Do not hold your breath; let it flow relaxingly. Make sure that your doctor agrees with your fitness program before you perform the aerobic or anaerobic exercises.

Muscular strength will help stop osteoporosis with routine exercises of your muscles and your bones. The body's skeleton stays stronger as the heart's efficiency increases. Mobility tones your muscles, improves your strength, strengthens the immune system, and shapes the body. You get better relaxation and gain good sleeping habits. Your exercises do not have to be vigorous but should be consistent for each repetition. Always start slow and build the muscles gradually by increasing stress in your exercises as you go along. For example, you might begin with two different aerobic exercises in a day and two times a week with 10-20 repetitions. As you master them you may include many different aerobic or anaerobic exercises.

Physical activities need not be exhaustive for your physique. The objective of fitness exercises is for your body to stay healthy as long as there is life in you. Create an environment that will keep your interest continuously as your condition, exercise level, and activities program improves. You will choose to conduct these exercises throughout your life.

Love   Live   Laugh

Your objective may be different if you are an athlete, where power exercises and anaerobic exercises are more predominant. Make sure that anaerobic exercises consist of lower repetitions depending upon the stress on your muscles. Repetitions depend upon your physical condition as an athlete.

This section covers the understanding of your body and helps you to design and enhance activities involving aerobic exercises. You will evaluate how much muscular exercise your body can handle to keep your health.

Do not ignore the health of your eyes. To maintain your eyesight, exercise the muscles of your eyes. All breathing exercises are related to improving your cardio-respiratory capacity and must be practiced to strengthen your lungs.

Abdominal and oblique exercises are included so you can maintain your body's contours—lean and mean. It is up to you to keep your body flexible, shapely, and ache-free with the help of these exercises.

Learn to massage your body or your partner's body muscles to reduce stresses and pains (refer Chapter: 'Massaging Your Body'.)

During the spring and fall many of us are confronted by seasonal allergies. It is important to avoid, as much as possible, exposure to these airborne allergens; therefore, the book provides a methodology for managing common allergies such as pollen.

I find that sleeping is a common problem, especially with our older generation. When you are worried or thinking about certain plans you may not be able to sleep easily. The book uses meditation techniques to overcome such problems.

Chapter 9

Physiology and Anatomy of the Human Body

The information in this chapter is for additional information. If you are not interested in learning about your body and the ligaments, you may skip this chapter.

The human upper body structure, as we observe in the illustration, from top to bottom consists of the brain (skull), the neck (cervical), the shoulders, the arms (humerus, radius and ulna) including the hands and fingers (metacarpal bones and phalanges), the rib cage of the chest holding our lungs and heart, and the spine (vertebral column) to support the body.

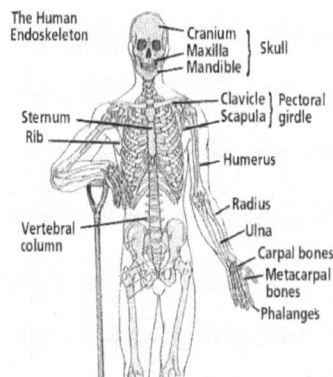

The lower body structure contains legs and knees (femur, fibula, tibia, patella, tendons, cartilage, and ligaments).

Love   Live   Laugh

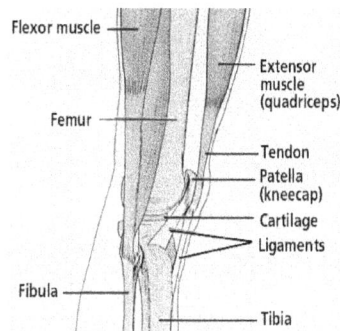

The feet and anklebones are tarsals, metatarsals and phalanges. These are all part of the human body, including the bones to support this structure. The blood flows through the passages of veins and arteries. Our body's support system does not consist of only the bones; it is much more complex than that. It includes ligaments that give the joints and muscles their movements. The digestive system of our body includes the intestines, the gallbladder, the liver and much more. Some functions related to the system are described below.

Energy for the muscles is supplied by the food we eat and the oxygen we inhale. For energy, the body initially uses sugars, and for additional energy it uses body fats as a supplement. The muscle fibers rely on the oxidative system for their energy. The oxidative system enhances during low intensity workouts. Neurotransmitters use energy and the muscles consume sufficient oxygen during low intensity exercises.

Neurotransmitters are needed to flex the muscles and maintain mental focus. Depletion of these can lead to fatigue, decreased performance, or even depression. The body needs some carbohydrates and essential fatty acids. A deficiency of either can cause health problems.

Exercise type, repetitions, and repetition speed will set the tempo for the activities you do. Structurally, each muscle is a bundle of muscle fibers that are essentially composed of proteins, myosin, and actins. The muscle fibers line up in a specific order as they contract. To maintain the muscles in that fiber-order, they need to be trained regularly. The muscles get trained depending upon the number of sets, the intensity, and the technique that you use.

Always, rest between exercise sets to avoid injury or overstressing your body. Since muscle fibers are dynamic, mix different exercises in your routine to achieve the maximum benefit in terms of your strength and endurance.

Brain – The brain works to analyze information before it transmits messages to various parts of the body. It works like a computer in which all decisions are made depending upon the information it receives from many different body sensors. It coordinates learning, memorizing, and analyzing your thoughts. Information and decisions are created and are then transmitted in bi-directional ways via the neurons.

Neck – The cervical vertebrae, which are part of the spine, form and control the movements of the neck. Its functions enable lateral and rotary movements. The neck supports the weight of the head and provides a passage for all nerves to transmit signals, and blood vessels for blood circulation between the brain and rest of the body. It also provides a nerve pathway for the respiratory and alimentary systems, like a conduit, while protecting the spinal cord.

Shoulder – The shoulder is the most mobile and flexible joint in the body. The muscles, tendons, and ligaments of the shoulders allow you to move and control your upper arm movements.

Arms – The function of the human arm is to enable you to reach, touch, and feel objects. The deltoid muscles help you lift your arms. The hands and fingers are moved by the flexors and extensors in the wrist and the fingers. All the sensed information is transmitted to the brain resulting in appropriate decisions and actions.

Ribs – The body cage is a formation of ribs to protect the inner organs. It maintains the shape of the body and its structure by forming your chest. Behind the cage the lungs and heart are located and are protected by this bone formation. The function of our lungs and heart keep us alive.

Lungs – The primary function of the lungs is to provide oxygen to the blood and remove carbon dioxide from it. The lungs accept incoming oxygen from the environment and give back toxins such as carbon dioxide and waste products of the body's cells. A lung works like a co-partner with the heart that is nestled over one corner on the left side of a lung, to transmit oxygenated blood to the heart.

Heart – The heart carries carbonated blood to the lungs and in exchange the oxygenated blood is returned to the heart. The heart delivers this oxygenated blood to every cell in the body, including the brain, to provide oxygen and nutrients. This process is called blood circulation. The heart has two pumps. Each has two muscular chambers. It is the contraction of these muscles that pumps the blood.

Spine – The spine provides strength and support for the human body. The major functions involve protecting the spinal cord and nerves, attaching the back muscles, providing back and body support, and providing the motion of the human skeleton – front, back, sideways and other options. The spine in an erect position with the head centered puts the vertebral column in the shape of the letter S. Neck to tailbone, the spine helps absorb shocks due to body movements. The S curve protects the vertebral column from breakage. It provides structural support for the head and chest by balancing the weight distribution.

Stomach and Digestive System – The stomach receives food and acts like temporary storage. The digestive parts that include the intestines, gallbladder, the pancreas and the liver change the food into a semi-liquid form. This semi-liquid food then passes through the intestines where various nutrients are extracted that are needed by the tissues for growth and energy. Some enzymes help the digestive system to extract nutrient components

Love   Live   Laugh

such as proteins, carbohydrates, and fat needed by the body. Unwanted materials are then eliminated, as well.

Legs, Knees and Ligaments – The leg muscles become the supporting base for all kind of movements—where the knee joins the femur (thigh bone), the tibia and the fibula (two bones of lower leg), and the patella (knee cap bone) that allows bending of the legs and provides side-to-side motions. The ligaments give stability to the knee and connect bone to bone.

Feet and Tendons – The feet provide a total base to support the body against gravitational forces. The tendons attach the muscle to the bone; the contracting motion of the muscle is transmitted through the tendon so that the respective bone or joint can move. Tendons help to hold the arch of the foot in its proper shape. The Achilles is a tendon of the calf muscle that is attached to the heel bone.

All of these body components are important for healthy living. Internal body components are equally important, if not more. This book is not meant to discuss the anatomy of the human body, but it gives just an overview to help you understand your body functionality.

Healthy living requires that all body components produce enough nutrients for your needs, their interaction with each other, muscle support of each region and their muscular strength. This book tries to cover all these factors and the health of these muscles.

Chapter 10

Aerobic Stretches

Who does not have a desire to look better, perform at a high level, feel healthier, and be more confident in engaging in a better quality of life? To accomplish all of these desires requires a comprehensive plan of physical activities in your daily routine, including:

1. Body flexibility and endurance of muscles

2. Conducting aerobic and anaerobic (if you can – not essential) exercises

3. Strengthening of muscles

4. Shaping your body to improve your looks

Muscle flexibility includes flexing and stretching muscles before starting any extensive exercise or other activity related to stretching. Aerobic exercises will increase your heart rate, your breathing rate, and the flexibility of your muscles. You can strengthen muscles with the use of elastic exercise bands or strings, and the application of breathing techniques. You can also lift small dumbbell weights in many different ways.

Some of the exercises I describe in this chapter are easy to do but I find them very helpful. Regularly doing stretching and breathing exercises will strengthen and lengthen your muscles to improve your body's flexibility. These exercises will also increase your range of motion and will be relaxing for your muscles.

Strong muscles will help you with exercises and will prevent injury to your body. Most basic stretching exercises can be performed at home without the need of any special equipment except a few stretchable bands or strings. Whenever you stretch your muscles, stretch them slowly and steadily with proper breathing and posture (refer Chapter 'Tips and Precautions'). Pay attention to the requirements of the exercise. Be careful not to push your muscles to the point of pain.

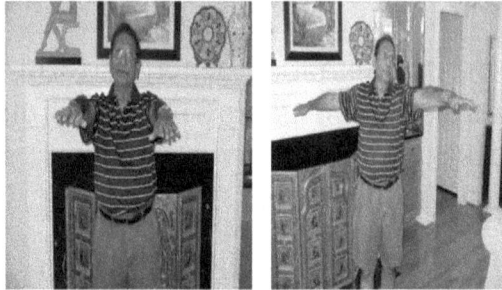

Stretching the Upper Body

- In a standing position, inhale and lift your arms in front of you. Hold your arms horizontal for a few seconds or to a count of ten. Exhale and bring your arms down to your sides. Repeat 10 times.

- Again, raise your arms in front of you, as above. Hold one arm horizontally in front while stretching the other arm to your side by twisting your oblique muscles and looking at the wall on the side of your twist. Twist as far as you can. Keep the twist for one second then return to your front. Twist the other side similarly. Repeat 3-5 sets. Bring your arms down by your sides.

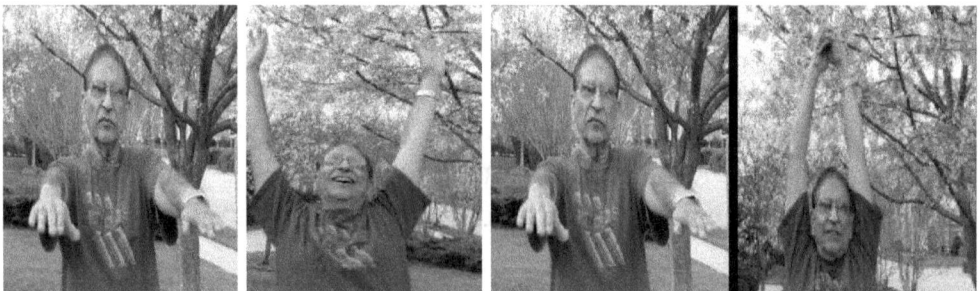

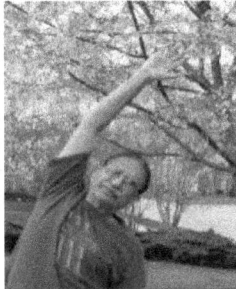

- Inhale and laugh loudly as you raise your arms parallel above and behind your head. Laugh as loud as you can. Exhale and return your arms to your sides. Repeat and laugh 10 times. This exercise is known as laughter yoga.

- Clasp your hands together above your head. Inhale and lift your arms as high as possible. Repeat 5 times.

- Lift one arm above your head while inhaling. Keep the other arm down at your side. Exhale and bend your body sideways to stretch your oblique muscles. Hold then return to the starting position while exhaling. Exhale as you bring your lifted arm back to your side. Repeat these steps for the other side to complete a set. Repeat 5-10 sets.

- Clasp both hands behind your back. Lift your clasped hands to stretch your biceps and shoulders. Repeat 5-10 times.

Stretching Your Calves

- Stand facing a wall. Place a support on the ground near the wall, approximately 2 inches high. Place the toes of one foot at the edge of this support and keep your heel on the ground. Your foot is angled. Lean against the wall with your palms on the wall thus transferring your body weight to the angled foot. Bend your knee a little towards

Love   Live   Laugh

the wall. Hold the stretch for a count of 35. Switch feet and repeat similarly, to complete a set. Repeat 5 sets.

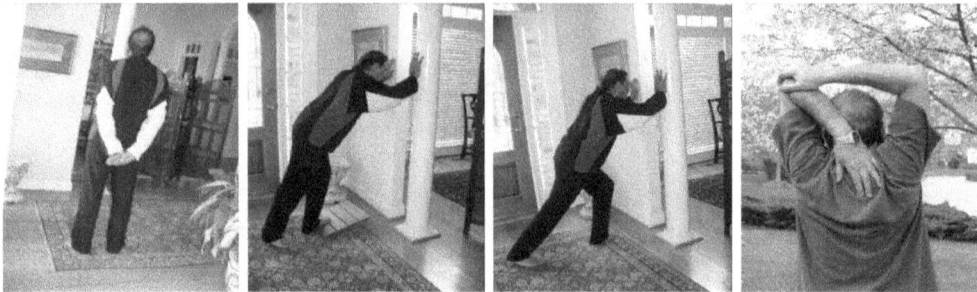

- Stand with your left foot in front of you and your knee bent slightly. Keep both feet flat on the floor. Lean against the wall. Feel pressure on your right calf. Hold this position for a count of 35. Switch feet and repeat similarly for the left calf. Repeat 5 sets.

- Bend forward with your hands on your knees. Lift your ankles to transfer your weight to your toes. Feel a stretch in your calves. Hold the stretch for a count of 5. Repeat 10 times.

- Lay flat on a surface. Stretch your legs with your toes pointing upward. Stretch your toes towards you. Your calves, thighs, and shin muscles will tighten. Hold the stretch for a few seconds then release. Repeat 5 times.

- Stretch your leg on a chair or on a bench. With the hand of your opposite side, try to reach your toes on the chair. The calf muscle of the leg on the chair will stretch. Hold; then switch legs to stretch the other calf. Repeat 5 times.

- If you use a stability ball, sit on the ball. Stretch both legs in front of you with your heels touching the floor and your toes pointing upward. Bend your knees and hold your toes. Now stretch your legs and toes away from the ball. Feel the stretch in your Achilles tendon. Repeat 2-3 times.

Relaxing Calf Muscles

Either while sitting on a stability ball or lying flat on a mat, stretch your toes towards you and away from you 3 to 4 times. It will relax your calf muscles.

Shoulders Stretches

- Lay flat on a surface with your arms by your sides and keeping your palms face up. Move both stretched arms simultaneously in a circular motion, rotating along your sides going towards and above your head. Inhale along with this movement. Make sure that your hands continue to keep in contact with the surface in this circular motion. With your hands behind your head, exhale and inhale a few times. Stretch both arms away from your head. Slowly reverse the movement of your arms, exhaling, to bring them back to your sides. Relax before repeating. Repeat 2-3 times.

- In a sitting or a standing position, place one hand between your shoulder blades. Hold its elbow with the other hand. Pull this elbow toward your head and let the hand resting between your shoulder blades slide down. This motion stretches the shoulder and the arm. Switch arms to repeat similarly. Repeat 5 sets.

Stretching your Back

- Stand with your feet slightly apart. Bend backward as far as possible. Maintain your balance during the bend. Hold this position for a count of 5-10. Return to your upright position. Repeat 5 times.

- Lay on a surface on your back bringing your feet near your buttocks. Raise both knees towards your chest by holding under the knees. Pull knees close to your chest. Hold this position for a 5-10 count. Repeat 5 times. This provides a stretch to the back and buttocks.

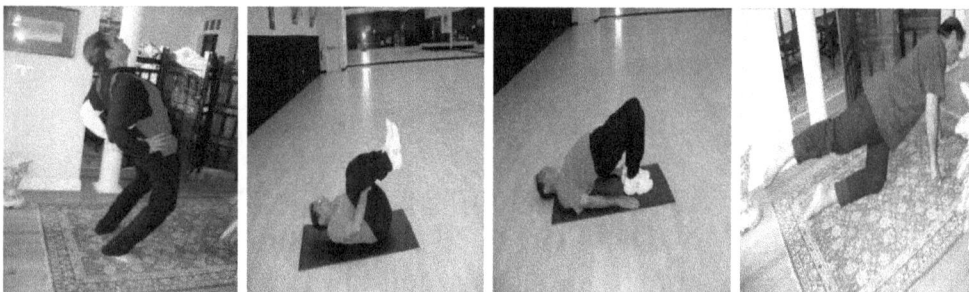

- Lay on a surface, as above, with your feet close to your buttocks and flat on the surface. Stretch your hands next to you or behind your head. Lift your buttocks while exhaling. Hold for a count of 5. Repeat 5 times.
- Curl your legs under you and sit on them. Bend forward to place both palms on the floor or mat. Lift your body and balance on your knees and palms. Stretch one leg backward, raising your foot as high as you can. Hold for a count of 5. Switch legs to stretch similarly for a set. Repeat 10 sets.

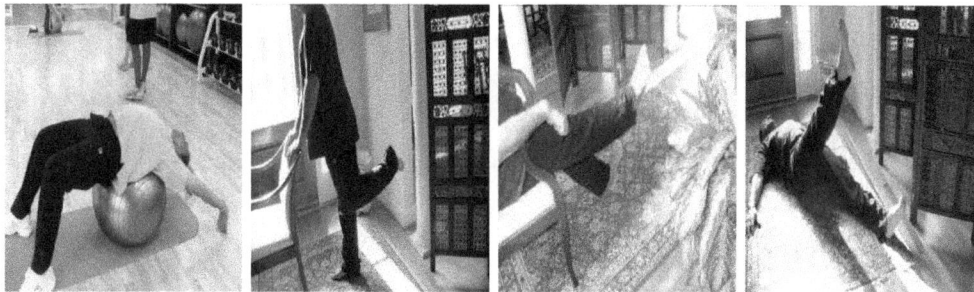

- Lay on a stability ball with your feet flat on the floor. Let your hands go behind your head and along the ball. You will stretch your back and spine by rolling along the ball. Stretch your legs and maintain your balance on the ball. Repeat two times.

Stretching your Thighs and Hips

- Hold and stand behind a chair. Move back a little and lift one leg backward bending the knee slightly. Lift the knee high towards your back as far as you can. Hold for a count of 5 then switch legs. Repeat similarly for a set. Repeat 5 sets.
- Sit in a chair with your one leg outstretched. Exhale and lift one leg as high as possible. Hold for a count of 5. Lower the leg while inhaling. Switch legs and repeat similarly. Repeat 5 times.
- Lay on your back with your hands by your sides. Stretch your legs on the floor or on a mat. Exhale and lift one leg above the ground as high as possible. Hold for a count of 5 then lower your leg to the floor while inhaling. Switch legs to repeat. Repeat the set 5 times.
- Sit on the floor or a mat with your feet touching each other, as shown. Pull the feet close to you. Place your arms on your knees to push your knees towards the floor. Feel pressure in your thighs. Repeat two times.

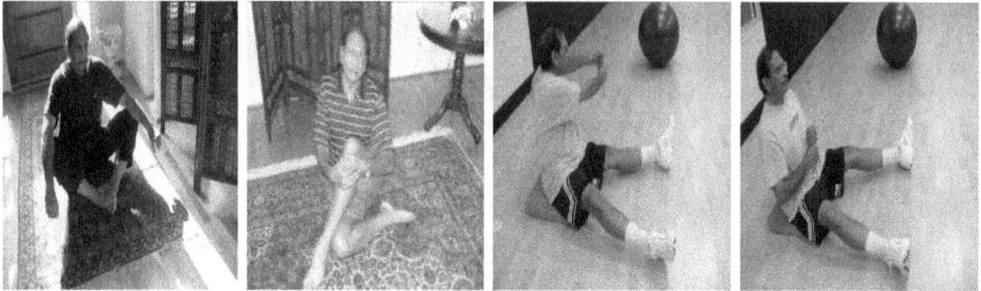

- Place your right foot across your left thigh or knee so that it is close to your hip. Place both hands on your right knee and pull your knee towards you (Note: right foot touches the surface). Feel a stretch in your right thigh, hip and oblique. Switch legs to repeat similarly. Repeat 5 sets.

Combining Multiple Stretches in One Exercise

Abdomen Exercise (Chakki Rotations)

Stretch your legs out, in front of you, on a floor. Hold one small bar, or a ball, or a piece of wood in your both hands. Stretch your arms in front of you. Pull your bellybutton inward. Rotate your hand together, keeping your arms outstretched, all the times, in your front and by your sides. Bend backward as hands come closer to you.

Pull your bellybutton inward. Stretch your hands horizontally as far away from self. First rotate *clockwise* the held object allowing your body to bend forward, to the side, backward and then rotate counter-clockwise, the other direction. Always keep your bellybutton pulled inward during each circular rotation. Rotate both, *clockwise* and *counter-clockwise* for 5 or more times.

(Note: in front you may bend elbows as if you are pulling an object).

This exercise will stretch your upper body, arms, obliques, and your abdomen. Stretch your breathing with your inhalations and exhalations. You may repeat this exercise more than 5 times.

You may use one hand at a time for the rotations. The rotations will not alter; However, using both hands gives more exercise to the whole body.

Drum Beat Exercise

This exercise takes care of multiple ailments. It strengthens your abdomen, pelvic and sphincter muscles.

Exercise – Exhale and pull-in your bellybutton, inhale and release your bellybutton

While holding your breath, release your bellybutton. Continue to pull-in then release your bellybutton thereby pulling and releasing abdominal muscles using a steady rhythm like a sound of a drum beat. Do it for a maximum period, for as long as you can comfortably hold your breath.

Do this rhythm often and several times to strengthen your muscles.

Chapter 11

Eye Exercises

Whenever you hear about exercising your body muscles you rarely think about exercising the muscles of the eyes. In fact, I have never heard anyone talk about exercising the eye muscles. Eyes are an essential and integral part of your body. Eyes are essential for your visual senses. You need to pay special attention to the muscles of your eyes.

Eyes contribute a very large part to our senses and our knowledge. People should get their eyes examined regularly to catch an early stage of any disease, especially glaucoma. Glaucoma damages the optic nerve in the eyes and can lead to loss of vision when it is not treated in time. Read more on this subject in National Eye Institute (NEI) documents. [The NEI is a division of the National Institute of Health (NIH)].

To keep eyes healthy you should take care of the eye muscles. Eye exercises energize the eye muscles. Eyes are the "camera" of our body; they activate our senses and transmit information to our brain cells on a consistent basis. Eyes are a sensitive part of our body that provides information for our enjoyment and happiness.

The eyes are the second most complex organ of our body next to our brain. The eyes are composed of more than two million working parts. Eyelids protect eyes by shielding them from intense light and the impact of foreign particles. Tears lubricate and nourish the eyes. Every time we blink, our eyelids act like windshield wipers to lubricate them. Six muscles control such movements. These muscles set all the other eye muscles in motion instantaneously for our vision.

Love   Live   Laugh

Eyes are the only part of our body that can function at any time during the day or the night. They help the arms, legs, and other body parts. Eyes are protected by the eyelids especially when they are resting.

Let your ophthalmologist examine your eyes from time to time to catch eye disorders; make corrective diagnoses of the blood vessels, optic disc, or refraction errors; and determine the general health of your eyes, including any foreseeable eye problems. Ophthalmologists are medically trained to diagnose and correct problems of the eyes.

Exercising, for strengthening your eyes, is essential and should be a very important part of your daily life.

Eye exercises helps:

- Expand the scope of your vision to be as wide as possible allowing you to see far and wide in different directions.

- Distinguish between the various colors in the environment surrounding you.

- Delay the formation of cataracts due to aging.

- Strengthen the eye muscles by increasing your concentration.

- Save the eyes from macular degeneration, or at least help reduce its effect.

- Maintain your retina's cone cells, rod cells, and fovea, where visual images are transmitted to the brain via your optic nerve.

Eye exercises may not fix existing problems but they are essential so that the eye muscles stay healthy throughout your life. I recommend that you exercise your eyes at least once a week. You can exercise more often as you like.

Love   Live   Laugh

Macular degeneration is an age-related degeneration. It is a common eye disease that causes deterioration of the macula, the central part of the retina, which is a paper-thin tissue at the back of the eye where light-sensitive cells send visual signals to the brain. Sharp, clear, straight-ahead vision, color and fine detail are processed by the macula. Damage to this part of the eye will result in blind spots or blurred or distorted vision. When the macula is damaged, many daily activities become increasingly difficult. To keep eyes healthy, relax the eye muscles. Blinking of eyelids or closing the eyes provides such relaxation. In addition, eye muscles replenish rest to the eyes. Eye drops, when applied, provide external lubrication to the eye muscles.

Eye Exercises to Maintain Healthy Vision

The eye exercises I describe here require you to keep your head steady and look ahead without bending or moving your head. Only your eyes should move during the exercises.

Exercise 1 - (Helps the concentration and focus of the eye muscles.)

1. Hold a finger at arm's length in front of you.
2. Concentrate on this finger without moving your head.
3. Start bringing the finger slowly towards you. Keep your concentration on the finger.
4. At a certain point, you may start seeing a double image of your finger. Stop your finger there. (It is possible that you may never see double image, meaning your eye muscles are fine.)
5. Return the finger to your arm's length again.
6. Repeat 10 times.

Love   Live   Laugh

7. Blink your eyes after each try to release pressure on your eyes.

8. Repeat 2-3 sets in a week.

Exercise 2 - (Helps peripheral concentration.)

In this exercise you will rotate your eyes along the periphery of your vision, stretching the muscles of the eyes. This exercise helps to maintain your eyes' side vision. Move your eyes in a clockwise circular rotation and then in a counter-clockwise circular rotation. Note that your head stays motionless and level.

1. Keep your head stationary, looking straight ahead.
2. Look up towards the ceiling, and stretch your vision upward.
3. Look down to aim your sight downward.
4. Repeat steps 2 and 3, 2 to 4 times.
5. Look towards your extreme right and stretch your vision by widening your eyes.
6. Look to your extreme left.
7. Repeat steps 5 and 6, 2 to 4 times.
8. Look at a 45-degree angle upward to the right stretch your vision.
9. Look at a 45-degree angle downward to your left.
10. Repeat steps 8 and 9, 2 to 4 times.
11. Look at a 45-degree angle left upward and stretch your vision.
12. Similarly, look downward and to the right at a 45-degree angle.
13. Repeat steps 11 and 12, 2 to 4 times.

After completing these steps, blink your eyes. Next start rotation of your eyes clockwise 2 to 3 times, and then rotate them in counter-clockwise 2 to 3 times.

Note: *Hold your head stationary and level at all times.*

Love   Live   Laugh

At the end of all these vision stretches, blink your eyes again to release pressure on the eye muscles. Rub your palms together to warm them and place them on your eyes lids for a few moments.

Eye Irritation

Redness is a sign of eye irritation. This condition might require consultation or treatment by your ophthalmologist or an emergency service. While waiting, my two suggestions below might provide some relief.

1. Apply over-the-counter eye drops. The eye drops will lubricate your eyes muscles. After the application, keep your eyes closes for a few minutes to relax them.

2. You may also use 1-1.5% Boric Acid Sterilizing solution. It may be available in your drug store. Generally, the boric acid bottle comes with an eyecup. Fill the eyecup with this boric acid solution and blink your eye in the liquid for half a minute. Wash the cup with tap water before you use it for your other eye. Your eyes may feel less irritated for a short time.

Success Stories

Since the eyes are one of the most precious organs of the body, use common sense to help save your sight.

In a gym, I saw a 14-year boy rubbing his eyes. A man standing next to him was telling him to continue rubbing his eyes. He thought it might help the boy with his eye irritation.

I approached the boy and asked him if he was wearing contact lenses. He was wearing contact lenses. I stopped him from rubbing his eyes and asked him if he had his eye drops so that he could apply the drops. He did not bring his eye drops that day. I suggested that he take a drop of tap water with the tip of his finger and apply it to his eye, allowing the water to drip from his finger to his eye a few times. He listened to me and applied the water. As suggested, he blinked his eyes after each application. His eye irritation stopped.

- A friend's wife was visiting us when she felt irritation in her eyes. I offered her boric acid solution to wash her eyes. She washed her eyes and felt better. (I use boric acid solution for my own eyes whenever I feel eye irritation.)

Chapter 12
Breathing Techniques

Our respiratory system gathers oxygen from the environment and processes it, then passes oxygenated blood to the heart. The heart delivers oxygen to the tissues of our body in the form of oxygenated blood. Body cells use the oxygen and produce carbon dioxide making deoxygenated blood, which is returned back to the right atrium of the heart. The deoxygenated blood is transported to our lungs for purification and re-oxygenated. The lungs will remove carbon dioxide and other toxins, which are exhaled into the environment.

Proper breathing is an important part of healthy existence. This includes breathing during exercise. Breathing will help relax the brain and body muscles. During breathing exercises, concentrate on the positive aspects of your surroundings. Correct body posture is essential to reduce strains and pain of the neck, spinal cord, back, and shoulders. Correct posture also facilitates the proper alignment and function of the spinal cord nerves that communicate with the brain.

Start inhalations and exhalations at a slow rhythm before starting exercises stretching of your muscles. An exercise routine will raise your breathing rhythm and the rate of your lung movement. The change of rhythm is considered normal as long as you do not become uncomfortable. If your breathing rate gets excessively high, take small breaks to restore more normal breathing and to get comfortable again. Regardless of your breathing rate, you should rest between stretches. It allows your muscles to recoup and reduces your muscle tension. Take a deep breath before lifting weight. When you are exercising to build muscle, or during anaerobic exercise, the inhalation and exhalation of deep breaths, help to relax your muscles at a much faster rate.

Love   Live   Laugh

Deep breathing means taking in a lot more oxygen. It is the oxygen therapy to boost the oxygen level in your blood stream. Muscles use oxygen efficiently and convert it to increase energy in your body, control your blood pressure, moderate cholesterol levels, and improve your physical fitness so you stay healthy. Such improved physical condition will make you feel more energetic.

Let us evaluate different breathing techniques to learn the specific steps for doing them. Breathing expands lung muscles. Expanded and strong lungs will intake more oxygen to the body. Extra oxygen will energize brain cells and remove toxins and carbon dioxide from the body so it functions efficiently. Knowing the health benefits, you are encouraged to implement these techniques in your daily life as much as possible each day.

The brain uses 40-50% of the oxygen that you inhale.

Yoga exercises utilize many breathing techniques and claim that proper breathing will not only keep you in good health but will also cure many ailments. The guidelines in this book may not match entirely with Yoga methods. Follow the techniques I describe depending upon your health and your body condition.

Breathing can be categorized into four areas: **upper body breathing, lower body breathing, alternate breathing,** and **deep breathing**.

Upper body breathing helps expand, stretch, and strengthen your lungs. Stronger lungs help to manage your breathing capacity. Upper body breathing is considered to be shallow breathing. It is shallow since it does not bring in enough air for the needs of the rest of your body. During upper body breathing, you pull your bellybutton inward during your inhalation. The inhaled air stays in your lungs to allow expanding and strengthening of your lungs. Pulling your bellybutton inward during your inhalation stops air from going to your belly.

This practice of pulling the bellybutton inward is done only in upper body breathing.

Lower body breathing encompasses routine type of breathing. You will inhale a higher amount of air (oxygen) to your system. This is also called diaphragmatic breathing. It keeps the tissues of your whole body healthy. In lower body breathing, you let your bellybutton go out during your inhalation and get pulled back during your exhalations.

Deep breathing helps remove immediate stress and expels a higher amount of toxins from the body. Oxygen intake during deep breathing increases to its highest limits.

Alternate breathing is related to energizing the mental lobes. It alternately energizes the right side, then the left side of your brain.

All above breathing exercises are simple and doable. You will gain insight to these breathings and their nature.

The Mayo Clinic handbook writes that our lungs, blood vessels and heart work together. The lungs receive oxygen from the environment and oxidize our blood. Our heart will pump the oxygenated blood to our arteries via the aorta that supplies oxygen and other nutrients to our body tissues. Forty to fifty percent of oxygenated blood goes to our brain. Our veins return deoxygenated blood to our heart for oxidation. This blood is recycled back to our body after our lungs oxidize it. Lungs remove carbon dioxide and other toxins from the received blood. Breathing exercises increase oxygen amounts in the blood thereby enhancing and purifying gaseous exchange processes. Since our lungs are so active, proper breathing techniques are an important part of maintaining good health.

When you combine your breathing with meditation, your stress level goes down. In meditation, it is suggested that you concentrate your attention on your breathing and keep your eyes closed. This helps to reduce distraction from your surroundings. Maintain good posture and enjoy some soft music in the background. Inhaling and exhaling through the nostrils is natural and is the most preferred method with some exceptions. These exercises, practiced often, can provide quality breathing and a healthy life.

Generally, lower body and deep breathing provide more relaxation to the body. Lower body breathing is diaphragmatic breathing (as mentioned earlier). The diaphragm is a dome-shaped muscle that separates the chest cavity from the abdominal cavity. If you place your finger just below your ribcage, you will feel diaphragm movements during your breathing. Diaphragmatic breathing provides an efficient exchange of oxygen and carbon dioxide with minimal effort. For example, during a baby's growth years, the baby's system automatically implements lower body breathing. We use lower body breathing as our normal breathing cycle especially during sleeping and resting periods. During lower body breathing, our abdominal area will expand and contract as we inhale and exhale.

For exercise purposes, lower body breathing is further enhanced to deeper breathing. In deep breathing, you hold your breath for much longer periods after each inhalation. The aim of deeper breathing exercises is to gather maximum toxins by air retention in your system. You discard maximum toxins during your next exhalation. This will increase the oxygen level in your body and the purification of your blood.

To summarize, the benefits of deep breathing include:

1. Providing a maximum supply of oxygen to the body.
2. Additional time to gather more toxins and waste.
3. Higher level of blood oxidation.
4. Breath retention increases lung elasticity and the capacity to be more powerful.

Love   Live   Laugh

During regular exercises, you may feel exhausted and may inhale or exhale at a much faster rate than normal, sometimes even profusely. Practice for longer periods inhaling through your nostrils and exhaling quickly through your mouth. This practice will bring your breathing to a normal rate.

Posture for Breathing Exercises

As mentioned earlier, optimal posture means keeping your spine erect at all times. During your breathing exercises, you may sit in a chair or on the floor, whichever is comfortable to you. No matter where you sit or stand, continue to pay attention to your posture. Do not let your back sag or head tilt. Your hands may relax in your lap or may be kept by your sides. Your posture is important since all your electrical impulses and chemicals (chemicals flow from the spine to the brain freely via neck nerves in the back), and communication travel from your spine to your brain and vice versa. The oxidized blood to your brain also travels through the same route. All these provide energy to your body.

Upper Body or Chest Breathing

Pulling of the bellybutton inward is used entirely for upper body breathing. It will raise your ribs, collarbone and shoulders as you inhale. Upper body breathing requires you to concentrate as you pull your bellybutton inward and your chest bulges out. You will avoid bulging of your abdominal area.

If you have breathing problems, do not practice this breathing exercise. If you have chest pain, reduced blood pressure, or signs of feeling drowsiness call your doctor or 911. Generally drowsiness is a sign of less blood flow to your brain.

Upper body breathing exercises may help to reduce asthma. Breathing with COPD (Chronic Obstructive Pulmonary Disease) can be managed to reduce flare-ups or exacerbations. Flare-ups can be triggered by respiratory infections, shortness of breath, or pollution. Long inhaling of fresh air takes in as much air as you can breathe with a single breath. You may try to exhale your breath by making a few short exhalations.

In addition to inhaling, the lungs also extract carbon dioxide or toxins from the returned blood and expel it to the atmosphere. As your lungs get stronger and healthier, your health will get better. Upper body breathing exercise helps your lungs get stronger. Your survival depends upon the efficiency of your lungs.

Upper body breathing is designed so that the larger percentage of air remains in the lungs and above – reaching only the pulmonary functions. The upper lobes of the lungs in a human's body have a very small air retention capacity. When a dramatic condition occurs, such as asthma or a cough, your body automatically switches your inhaling to upper body breathing.

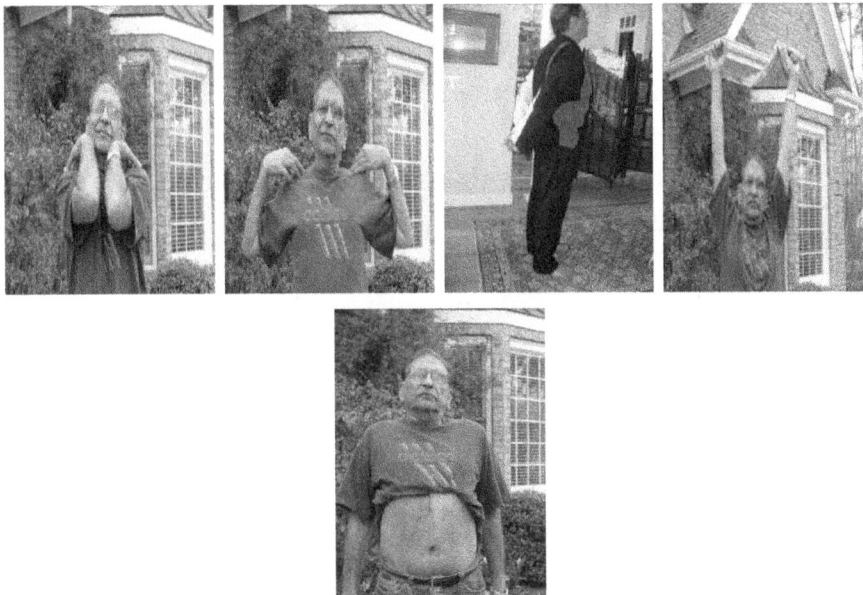

Upper Body Breathing Exercises

- Place your hands over your shoulders and inhale while pulling in your bellybutton. Squeeze your elbows together in front of you during your exhalation. Your elbows may touch each other. Next, stretch your elbows backward and inhale. Again, pull in your bellybutton. Hold your position and count to 10 before exhaling. Repeat these steps 10-15 times. Repeat 2 to 3 sets.
- Raise your fists at your chest level with your thumbs directed upward. Inhale slowly and pull your stomach inward and your fists to your sides. Exhale and bring your fists in front of your chest, releasing your stomach. Repeat this step 10 to 15 times. Repeat 2 to 3 sets.
- Start with your both hands resting on your shoulders. Keep your stomach pulled-in during this exercise. Lift both your arms parallel and upward above your head while inhaling and exhaling at a rapid speed. Exhale to bring your hands down to your shoulder. Your hand movements up and down should be fast during this exercise. Repeat these actions 20 to 30 times or more. Repeat 2 to 3 sets.
- In this exercise, your stomach will move in and out by pulling in your bellybutton while inhaling, and by releasing your bellybutton as you exhale. You inhale and exhale at a faster speed and your bellybutton will move in and out at about the speed of a drumbeat. You will inhale and exhale 40 to 50 times (or more) in a sequence without slowing or stopping. Relax for a few minutes then repeat the same sequence as many times as you can.
- Your arms and hands are relaxed and by your sides. Exhale and bend your chin down so it almost touches your chest. Inhale quickly by pulling your abdomen inward then raise your head. Repeat inhalation and exhalation 20 to 30 times. Do 2 to 3 sets.

If you feel dizzy during any step, stop and do not continue.
Relax and return to your normal breathing.

Breathing Exercise for your Relaxing

Breathing normally, brings your hands in front of your chest. Hold them together. Lift both your hands above your head while inhaling. Bring your hands down by your sides while exhaling. Repeat 5 times. Now reverse the movement of your hands and arms. Inhale and lift your hands by your sides for them to meet above your head. Hold your hands together there and bring them together in front of your chest while exhaling. Repeat 5 times. Your breathing will return to almost normal.

Lower Body Breathing

Lower body breathing utilizes all the channels of your body, including the chest and abdomen. This technique uses your abdomen to store air temporarily. Your chest muscles move to control your lungs. In normal breathing, you automatically adapt to lower body breathing. When you wear a tight belt or when your stomach is full or when you are feeling short of breath, lower body breathing will help you to return to normal.

Lower body breathing takes in maximum oxygen from your lungs, as your heart circulates the oxygenated blood to your body via your aorta. The oxygenated blood is distributed to your body's lymph system.

If you are breathing heavily due to fatigue or a problem, implement Relaxed Breathing Technique, described above.

Reminder: Always maintain your posture during breathing exercises.

Love   Live   Laugh

This breathing is a diaphragmatic breathing and it distributes the inhaled air. These exercises fill your lungs and stomach with air rather than only your lungs as was in the case of upper body breathing. The presence of the extra air in the body allows a higher level of blood oxidation thus increasing its purification. Physically, your stomach will expand, get larger, during your inhalation and will return to normalcy during your exhalation.

Lower Body Breathing Exercises

- Inhale slowly and raise both hands above your head. Hold for a count of 10. Exhale all your breath as fast as you can and move your hands to your shoulders. Your abdomen will return to its original position. You will exhale carbon dioxide to the environment. Repeat 20 to 25 times. Repeat the set again.

- Place both hands on your shoulder blades (top back) with your elbows pointing upward. Inhale and allow your stomach to expand normally. Move your elbows outward. Exhale and bring your elbows closer. Pull-in your bellybutton. Repeat 20 to 25 times. Repeat the set again.

- Place both hands on your waist. Inhale normally while pulling your elbows backward, then exhale slowly with elbows returning and your bellybutton pulled inward. Repeat 20 to 25 times. Repeat the set again.

- Hold both hands with your fingers clasped behind your back, stretching your arms. Inhale normally while lifting your hands upward as far as you can. Exhale and release the stretch and pull your bellybutton inward. Repeat 20 to 25 times.

Deep Breathing Exercises

Deep breathing is an extension of lower body breathing. With deep breathing, you will inhale over longer periods; you will hold the inhalations for as long as possible, and then exhale by pulling your bellybutton inward. You may bend forward during your exhalation to release a maximum amount of carbon dioxide. During your exhalations you may apply light hand pressure to your abdomen, pressing it inward. Exhale a few times to release maximum carbon dioxide. This will result in maximum inhalation of oxygen in your next round of breathing with your upright posture. Repeat these steps 3 times.

This scenario of inhalation and exhalation I have described will let you inhale additional oxygen compared to your ordinary inhalation. It will also allow you to exhale more toxins and carbon dioxide during each exhalation. Never press your abdomen hard with your hands.

Deep breathing is also a part of diaphragmatic breathing. These breathing cycles will provide a higher level of oxidation to your blood. It will also improve your health. Deep breathing is a healthy exercise. You should practice deep breathing often or at least once a day. During this exercise, concentrate on your breathing. Keep yourself calm and relaxed, similar to meditation.

Alternate Nostril Breathing

As the name implies, in this exercise you breathe through one of your nostrils at one time then through the other.

You will start this exercise by inhaling through your left nostril and exhaling through your right nostril. Next you will inhale through your right nostril and exhale through your left nostril. After inhalation hold your breath for a count of 5-10. Your body should stay relaxed and you should pull in your bellybutton during your exhalation.

Love   Live   Laugh

Alternate Nostril Breathing Steps

Form a V-shape with your fingers. You may use any two fingers. In yoga exercises, your thumb and your pinky finger are used to form the V-shape. (When you use your thumb and pinky for the V-shape, your forefinger, middle finger and ring finger will rest on your forehead.) I use forefinger and middle finger of my hand to make a V-shape.

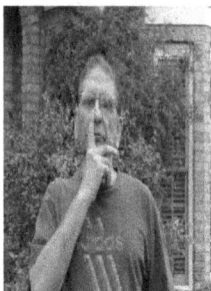

Consider you are using your right hand's thumb and pinky for a V-shape.

- Press your right nostril lightly with your thumb while your left nostril stays open for inhalation.
- Inhale through your left nostril and hold your breath. Switch to close your left nostril and release the right nostril to exhale then to inhale. Exhale via your right nostril and then inhale via your right nostril to hold your breath.
- Switch your fingers again to begin the next cycle. Each cycle is a round of inhalations and exhalations.
- Continue the rounds of inhalation and exhalation by switching nostrils. Repeat 5 to 10 rounds.

Love   Live   Laugh

Alternating nostril breathing can be practiced at any time and in any place. Moreover, the alternate nostril breathing exercise does not require your complete concentration, as was the case with other breathing exercises.

When you cannot practice your other breathing exercises, you may still complete your alternate nostril breathing exercise to maintain your health. Alternate nostril breathing will work to energize your brain lobes. It will increase your breathing capacity and give your breathing flexibility.

Benefits of Alternate Nostril Breathing (Yoga)

Alternate nostril breathing exercises energize both lobes of the brain, making them function more efficiently. The left-brain hemisphere controls the right side of your body functions and the right-brain hemisphere controls the left side of your body functions. Both lobes manage different types of information and actions (refer Chapter: ' Brain & Memory Simulation').

The Mayo clinic book says, "The two major areas [of the brain] are the cerebrum and the cerebellum." The speech, memory, and vision are controlled in the cerebral hemispheres. The right hemisphere of the brain, controls muscles of the left side of the body. The left hemisphere of the brain controls the muscles of the right side of the body. This appears to be a similar kind of division that is found in yoga literature.

The above relationship supports the alternate nostril breathing exercises that energize both sides of our brain. Alternate nostril breathing exercises will help you relax and help your nervous system to feel calm. For additional relaxation to your senses, rub your palms together to warm them, and then place your warm palms on your eyes for a few moments.

Caution: If your nostrils are congested or blocked, breathing exercises may not be suitable for you.

Love   Live   Laugh

If you sit in a steam room you may want to use Eucalyptus fumes. Ask the facility attendant for Eucalyptus crystals. Eucalyptus is known to reduce congestion. Eucalyptus is considered therapeutic for many respiratory systems, however not enough medical data exists for the American Medical Association to recommend it. Additionally, the FDA has not classified Eucalyptus as a drug. Check its side effects before using it.

Mixed Breathing Exercises

Stand straight and tall, with your shoulders leveled relaxed and your head straight. Start marching in place during these exercises as if you are in military.

- Start lower body breathing by inhaling, and lifting and stretching your hands in front of you at chest level. Rotate your arms by your sides. Turn your palms 180 degrees to face downward. Lower your arms to your sides while exhaling. Repeat a few times.
- Raise your arms by your sides. Turn your palms face down with your arms outstretched. Hold your arms level to your shoulders. Breathe normally as long as possible.
- Turn your palms upward, and then raise them above your head while inhaling and pulling in your bellybutton. Your palms will meet above your head. Bring both hands together in front of your chest exhaling to release pressure on your bellybutton. Repeat 10 times.

Chapter 13
Therapeutic Breathing

When you are in a good health, you will generally not give a second thought to your breathing capacity since the breathing and respiratory mechanisms of your body are a normal way of life. The oxygen that you inhale keeps your body tissues and all other parts of your body healthy.

Before incorporating therapeutic breathing exercises in your daily life, you should relax your body, brain, and all of your muscles. Lower body breathing as was described in earlier Chapter will help.

If you have a breathing problem, consider having your lung capacity checked using the Spirometry tests. Spirometry tests are generally conducted under the supervision of a pulmonary physician to determine the existence of COPD (Chronic Obstructive Pulmonary Disease). Your doctor may also ask for a CT scan if your condition warrants. The Spirometry tests are very simple. They involve blowing into a test tube while a technician measures your lung capacity. To do this, the technician will measure your inhalations and how fast you can blow out air (FVC). The measurements will also include how fast you can inhale and exhale over a predetermined period, generally over a one-second period (FEV1). FVC and FEV1 are compiled to determine the health of your lungs by comparing the results to a healthy person of the same height, age, sex, and race. If you need these tests, go to a pulmonary physician.

Most metabolic syndrome problems of the lungs are strongly linked with abdominal obesity where the breathing problems occur. Obesity should be checked to keep your metabolic condition at a healthy level. A three-inch increase in your waistline will increase your metabolic syndrome condition by 5 to 8 times. Metabolic syndrome has a link to an increase in blood pressure, blood sugar, and cholesterol. Body fats limit the expansion of the lungs and chest during your inhalations that may even cause inflammation that will make breathing more difficult.

What are the warning signs? They are wheezing, an increase in cough, chest tightness, or a drop in the peak flow meter reading. These signs may be due to your chest congestion or nasal flow. When a warning sign appears, relax to overcome the symptoms. A woman in my breathing and meditation class told me that her peak flow meter reading always had stayed consistent at 2.5, but it changed to 4.0 after following my 'Breathing and Meditation techniques', this was a good result.

Consider how the cooler temperatures irritate the lungs. Cold temperatures will send a signal to your nerves to reduce the intake of cold air. Your nerves will send signals to your lungs to constrict your airways thus causing a tightening or narrowing of your air passages to reduce an intake of cold air. This reduction of air intake will also reduce the available oxygen to your lungs. Oxygen availability may become insufficient for your body's needs. The process of restriction happens to all humans, whether they are in good health or have some breathing problem such as asthma or COPD. The reduction in your breathing capacity, if you are healthy, will not be felt since the percentage of reduction may not be enough to cause a problem because you keep meeting your body's needs.

However, when you have lower breathing capacity, even a small reduction of available oxygen will result in a high percentage of oxygen reduction for your body. Lower quantity of oxygen will affect your body functions more intensely.

This explains why asthma or COPD sufferers are advised to avoid cold atmospheres. The chilly weather will produce shortness of breath. To avoid a chill, wear a scarf around your exposed body including your face, head, and nose. Wearing warm clothes is essential. Cold weather should not restrict you from enjoying an outdoor life as long as you take precautions.

Love   Live   Laugh

Air get rarified at certain heights; for example, in high mountain ranges. The heights will produce shortness of breath due to reduced oxygen levels.

Therapeutic breathing exercises are different breathing exercises, compared to the breathing techniques discussed earlier. Therapeutic breathing exercises can help other breathing difficulties. An increase in your breathing capacity is good for your lungs and heart. All improvements take time to be effective. You must practice breathing exercises continuously

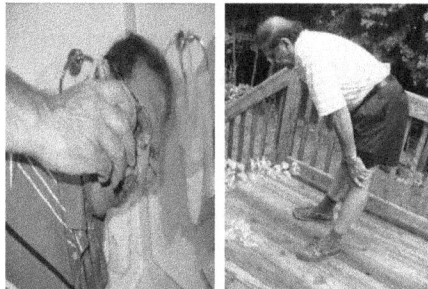

Therapeutic breathing exercises involve clearing your breathing and airways. For these exercises you may sit in a chair, sit on the floor, or you may stand in an optimal posture as described earlier in this book. If an exercise requires a different posture, that posture will apply only to that particular exercise.

- For therapeutic breathing exercises, clear your nostril airways by using a Neti-Pot. (Refer to Chapter: 'Managing Pollen & Allergies'.) The Neti-Pot package contains instructions for its use.

- Diaphragmatic breathing – The diaphragm is described as a dome-shaped muscle under the ribcage. Bend forward to move your diaphragm for an easy breathing. During your inhalation, space for air to enter the lower lobes of your lungs is created. Deeper inhalations will increase your diaphragmatic breathing. Repeat 10 to 20 times.

- Lie on your back and raise your backbone on several pillows, or by using hard foam under the middle of your spine. Place one hand on your chest. Inhale as much air as you can, allowing your belly to rise. The hand on your chest should not feel any movement. Exhale as you keep your hand on your chest. Make sure that your hand does not move up or down during your breathing cycles. Practice 20 times.

- Inhale slowly to take in as much air as you can, and then hold your breath for a count of 10. Exhale as fast as you can and press your abdominal muscles or bellybutton inward with light hand pressure to your abdominal muscles while exhaling. Repeat 30 to 50 times.

- Stand and bend with your hands over your knees. Tuck your chin to touch your chest. Exhale most of your breath. Pull in your bellybutton with the help of your abdominal muscles. Exhale more if you can. Hold your exhaled breath and rotate your stomach in a clockwise direction 2 to 3 times, then reverse the rotations of your stomach in a counter-clockwise direction 2 to 3 times. Take a deep breath, as you stand-up tall and high. Repeat these steps once again.

- In an optimal standing posture, raise both of your arms above your head as you inhale. Exhale your breath fast and bend forward at the same time. Your arms are pointing downward. Quickly raise your body upward while inhaling to a standing position. Your lungs are filled with fresh air. Bring your arms to your sides and exhale slowly. Relax a bit before repeating these steps. Conduct the same exercise 2 to 3 times for a set. You may repeat the set as many times as you like. If you get dizzy, stop the exercise.
- To manage a cough, sit relaxed in a chair. Cross your arms in front of you, just above your abdomen. Inhale slowly through your nose with your mouth closed. Now, curl your lips slightly and cough sharply two to three times through your mouth. Lean forward during your

coughing period and press your elbows gently against your abdomen. Return to an upright posture while inhaling. Release your arms and hold your breath for a short time before exhaling. Start the same repetition. Repeat 10-15 times. Repeat this set a few times as needed.

- To manage your mucus or lung secretion, inhale deeply through your nostrils. Hold your breath for a moment. Curl your tongue out and cough it out in 2 to 4 short coughs. Start your coughs from gentle to sharp cough. Repeat 5-10 times. Take a short rest then repeat the set.

If you feel dizzy during any exercise, STOP the exercise.

The therapeutic breathing exercises described here will provide oxygen to all of your body cells and lymph tissues and put you into a relaxed mood.

Chapter 14

Abdominal Exercises

Self-presentation is very important when you are making a first impression. In addition to other considerations, people will notice if you are lean, fit, and looking well. Many times, a fit and trim appearance can be a sign that you are capable of managing your actions. For your health, it is important for you to exercise and manage your diet so you look trim and healthy.

Being overweight can cause heart problems, high blood pressure, and high cholesterol levels. You can overcome these conditions.

The following exercises will help you to pull in your stomach muscles thereby making your abdominal area flatter. Oblique exercises will also help; these will be described in the following chapter.

The food that you consume goes into your stomach—a "storage area." Avoid exercises until the food gets digested. To avoid problems during abdominal exercises, I recommend that your stomach be nearly empty before exercising. When you get thirsty during exercises, quench your thirst with a few sips of water and it should not affect the abdominal exercises.

Before starting the abdominal exercises, conduct a few relaxation and stretch exercises. Many different exercises for the abdominal area have been published and are widely available through a variety of medias. Most exercises can be done at home. However, some exercises may require special machines. These machines are only available in health clubs or fitness facilities.

First two exercises can be done at home without the need of extra equipment. Other exercises you can also do at home ut requires a few inexpensive items. Where expensive equipment is needed, you may decide to go to a health club.

Exercise 1

1. Lay on your back on the floor or a mat.
2. Lift your feet up above your hips towards you.
3. Extend your hands towards your feet, trying to reach your toes.
4. Lift your shoulders and exhale to extend your hands and pull your abdominal muscles inward. Hold this stretched position for a count of 30.
5. Return your shoulders to the surface, inhaling before repeating the exercise.
6. Repeat 20-30 times.
7. Do 2-3 sets.

Exercise frequently until your stomach muscles attain the desired shape. Thereafter, you may reduce frequency of those exercises.

Exercise 2

1. Lay on your back on the floor or a mat.
2. Lift one foot and try to reach that foot with your opposite hand. Lift your shoulder and exhale to pull your stomach muscles inward. Change your feet and hands to repeat. Do the exercise in a fast motion.
3. Continue alternating feet and hands for 20 to 30 times per set.
4. Relax a little and repeat 2-3 sets a day. After achieving your goal, you may reduce the frequency to one set per week.

Love   Live   Laugh

If you have a stability ball, use it for the following exercises.

Exercise 3

1. Lay on the stability ball, on your back, keeping feet on the floor.
2. Inhale and hold and place your hands behind your head, shown above. You may hold a dumbbell with both hands.
3. Lift your hands above you lifting your shoulders exhale and pull your abdominal muscles inward.
4. Repeat 20-40 times in a set.
5. Do 2-3 sets each week.

Exercise 4

1. Lay on your back in the middle of a stability ball maintaining your balance.
2. Place your hands under your neck, as shown above.
3. Keep your knees and shoulders almost level, support your neck.
4. Lift your shoulders up 45 degrees and exhale pulling your abdomen muscles. This motion will tighten your abdomen and gluteus muscles. Lift your pelvis a little during the stretch.
5. Repeat 20-30 times in a set. Repeat the set 2-3 times per week.

Exercise 5

1. Lay on your back in the middle of a stability ball, holding manageable dumbbells in each hand or a medicine ball with both hands.

2. Stretch your arms, keeping them parallel to your right side shoulder. Exhale as you stretch and pull in your bellybutton inward. Roll stability ball to your left to twist your right oblique.

3. Repeat the sequence 10-15 times each side.

4. Relax before repeating the next set again.

Note: If you get a stomach cramp, abandon the exercise and recover your strength.

Chapter 15
Oblique Exercises

Trimming of the oblique muscles will help you to get back into shape. Your obliques are part of your abdomen. With a flat abdomen and trimmed obliques, you will look very sharp.

Notice that when you lift one of your arms above your head, your oblique muscle on that side gets stretched. Oblique exercises are based upon stretching your side muscles. To increase the intensity of the stretches, hold some manageable weights in each hand.

Exercise 1

1. Stand upright on the floor or a mat, with your feet apart equal to your body's width.
2. Hold manageable dumbbells in each hand.
3. Raise your right arm above your head and bend yourself toward your left.
4. Your right oblique side will get stretched.
5. Repeat 10-20 times.
6. Switch the dumbbells in your hands lifting your left hand above your head. Bend yourself toward your right side to stretch your left oblique.
7. Repeat 10-20 times.
8. Repeat 1-2 sets.

Love   Live   Laugh

In a gym or fitness center, this exercise can be done on an inclining machine by leaning your body in a tilted position, as below.

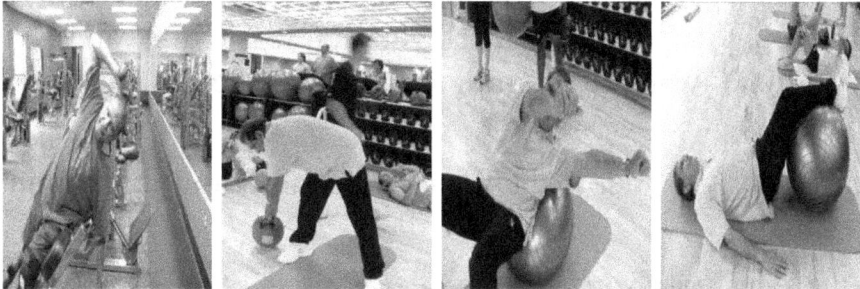

Exercise 2

1. Stand upright with your feet apart at body width.

2. Select a medicine ball weighing 5-10% of your body weight.

3. Exhale and draw your bellybutton inward, holding the ball in front of you.

4. Swing the ball to your right and place it on the floor, as shown. Return to an upright position and inhale.

5. Exhale and drawn in your bellybutton. Bend to lift the ball from the floor. Bring it to your front as you return again to an upright position.

6. With a scooping motion, swing the ball toward the left and exhale pulling-in bellybutton. Place the ball on the floor, then return to your upright position while inhaling.

7. Exhale and pull in your bellybutton to lift the ball to bring it in front of you.

8. Repeat the sequence 5-10 times. Do 1-2 sets.

Love   Live   Laugh

Exercise 3

1. Lay on your back on the floor or a mat, looking up.
2. Lift both legs above your hips.
3. Lift your right shoulder to reach your left leg. Exhale and pull your bellybutton inward as you lift the shoulder. Support your neck with both hands.
4. Return your shoulder to the floor and inhale. Your feet continue to stay lifted.
5. Do the same with your left shoulder. Remember to exhale and pull your bellybutton inward as you lift the shoulder.
6. Continue these stretches 10-20 times.
7. Relax after each set and before repeating the set.
8. Do 2-3 sets a day until you achieve your goal. Thereafter, you may reduce its frequency to one set in a week.

Exercise 4

1. Lay facing up on a stability ball. Hold a medicine ball in your hands.
2. Exhale and pull in your bellybutton, stretch your arms to your right side and roll the ball towards the left.
3. Twist your oblique.
4. Return your arms over your chest and repeat 10-15 times.
5. Repeat similarly for your left oblique, 10-15 times.
6. Repeat these steps once again.

Exercise 5

1. Lie on a mat with a stability ball under your legs.
2. Roll the ball to go from left to right directions and stretch your obliques.
3. Roll the ball 15-20 times.
4. Do 2-3 sets each time.

Exercise 6

This oblique exercise is called the "wood chop" exercise. Use a multi-purpose pulley machine for this exercise. Using both hands, you will pull a rope diagonally, from a position above your head, across your body and down towards your feet. Remember to exhale during the pull, draw your bellybutton inward, and twist your obliques. Set the pulley level at different heights, as shown in the photographs. Select a desirable and comfortable weight to pull with the rope.

1. Place the pulley at the top of the pole position.
2. Stand at the center of the multi-purpose machine with your feet parallel to your body width and facing say north. Pull the weights away from the stack. With your bellybutton pulled inward and your oblique twisted, repeat wood chops 10 times.
3. Turn to face to the south and repeat the wood chop at the same level 10 times.
4. Move the pulley to the mid-level of the pole. If needed, adjust the weight for your pull. Facing north, do wood chops 10 times.
5. Turn to face south and repeat wood chops at the same level, ten times.

6. Move the pulley to the bottom of the pole. Facing north, do wood chops by lifting your grip to the highest level, away from the weight stack, 10 times.

7. Turn to face south. Repeat wood chops at the same level, 10 times.

8. Repeat this entire sequence again.

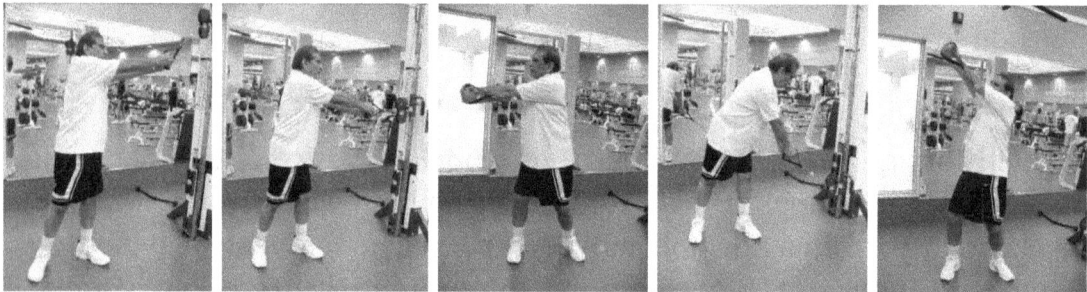

Exercise 7

1. Lay on your side on a mat and support your head.
2. Move your upper leg backward and forward, stretching it to go as far as possible.
3. Turn to exercise your other side.
4. Repeat each side 25-30 times.
5. Do 2-3 sets.

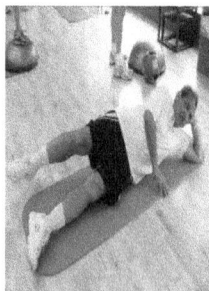

Love   Live   Laugh

Gentle Oblique Exercise Steps

To do this exercise, you may stand or sit, but feel yourself tall and high with an erect spine. Look straight ahead.

1. Raise both elbow with hands in front of you and inhale.
2. Bend to your left, raising your right elbow above your head. Breathe normally.
3. Rotate your upper body counter-clockwise exhaling and your bellybutton pulled in. Look toward the wall behind you.
4. Hold the twist to a count of 5 then return while inhaling.
5. Bring both elbows leveled and exhale.
6. Repeat similarly for the counter-clockwise side twist.
7. Repeat this sequence 5 times for both clockwise and counter-clockwise twists.

Chapter 16

Massaging your Body

Massage can be both stimulating and relaxing for your nerves, organs, muscle tone, and circulation. You massage your body by moving your palms and fingers in a circular motion. Always stroke toward your heart; this will prevent pushing your blood against the flow in your closed valves. Massage can be performed on the back, shoulders, arms, elbows, hands, the ridge of the skull, legs, feet, and even around your breasts. Massaging the temples reduces headache tension. You will need help for back massage.

Massager's palms and fingers will apply tolerable pressure during massage. To create more pressure, a massager may use both hands and her body weight. Use fingers to massage the neck area, and the fingers and palms to massage the spine area. The massager will massage vertebrae with fingers and will slide both palms from the spine and toward the sides of your back. The backs of your legs and its sides are massaged with the palms going downward toward the feet. It is possible to massage most of your own body yourself, but for unreachable parts you will need the help of another person.

Before a massage, select a quiet and serene environment where you will not be disturbed. Find sore spots on your body that need massage. When your massager is someone else, close your eyes and concentrate on your breathing during the massage. Let your body and mind feel relaxed.

Generally, body massages are conducted in a lying position on a massage bench or on a flat surface. The massager may warm up her palms by rubbing them together. She may apply some oil on her palms to apply it to the massage area. A massager's fingers, palms, and hands should move smoothly, with light pressure. She should have soft and relaxed hands and

Love   Live   Laugh

should maintain palm pressure during all the strokes. While slow massage movements relax the body, faster movements stimulate the muscles. Do not pause during the massage period. Massaging should be a continuous process. Oil is used to reduce friction between the hands and your skin to avoid frictional pain.

Back Massage

Lay on your stomach. All massage movements will go from your shoulder blades to the sacrum in the back. The massager applies gentle thumb pressure on both sides of the spine. She will knead along the edges of the spine with a small circular motion with her thumbs, kneading every vertebra joint deeply and gently. The massager will massage the back with both palms simultaneously for deeper work, covering one palm slide with the other palm slide. Her palms will move down the back avoiding pressure on the spine itself. The massage remains continuous and these steps are repeated a few times, going from light pressure to a successive increase in pressure. Light pressure is always applied to stiff and tender areas. After completion of the above steps the massager may tap the back slowly with the sides of her hands. She will shake the back muscles with her fingers to make the blood flow back to normal in the body.

Shoulder Massage

The massager will use thumb pressure over your shoulders, moving her thumbs from the neck joint to the shoulder area and toward the edges of the shoulder sides. This step will continue a few times, going from lighter pressure to a successive increase in pressure. The massager's hands move from the upper part of the back toward the sides of the shoulders. After a few rounds, shake the shoulder muscles to finish this area of massage. For this massage, the massager will slide palms from 1/3 below neckline along the spine to the edges of your shoulders to unwind strain in the shoulders.

Love   Live   Laugh

Neck Massage

Apply thumb pressure to both sides of the neck, massaging from the top of the neck toward the shoulder joints. Begin with light thumb or finger pressure (fingers are at right angle to your neck), and increase the pressure level along each slide. Slide the thumbs or fingers over the neck area as many times as needed.

Arm to Hand Massage

Massage one arm at a time. Start from the shoulder and move the palms and fingers in a rotating motion along the arm, elbow, the lower part of arm, the hand and fingers. The massager moves her hands along the upper and lower sides of the arm, the elbow, and the wrist. Both hands move simultaneously following each other for a continuous massage. Hands are massaged on both sides rubbing the hand from wrist to fingers, repeating a few times. The massager grasps each of your fingers and pulls and twists each finger gently. With a soft fist, she slowly taps the whole arm and shakes the arm with her fingers to energize the arm muscles.

Leg and Calf Massage

You will lie on your stomach. The massager should palpate the leg first to find some sore areas. Apply palm pressure from the foot to the top of the leg in a circular motion. Knead the legs and calves with full palm pressure. Repeat the palm movements from the feet to the top of the legs. After the massage, the massager will use the side of her hand to tap the legs and buttock with a fist. Shake the leg muscles with the fingers. Always reduce pressure over your knees and sore areas. Massage will help relax your joints, nerves, and the leg and calf muscles.

Place your foot on massager's shoulder, when massager is massaging the front of your leg. The massager will move towards you, building pressure in your thighs and knees. It will stretch leg muscles and will release your leg stress. Massage your leg by bending it at your knees towards your hips.

Foot Massage

Begin foot massage with warming strokes using the full palm on the bottom and top of each foot. The massager holds one heel at a time and makes a cup shape with her thumb and index finger, and her palm underneath. She rotates hand-made cup over your heel both clockwise and counter-clockwise directions for multiple rotations. She moves her palms over and under the foot from the heel toward the toes, massaging the foot. Next, the massager makes the cup again and rotates it over each toeyou're your heels in both directions. The massager will pull the toes slightly outward, stretching them gently to the point of resistance but twisting them to no more than a 90-degree angle. Complete the massage for each foot by massaging the upper and lower sides of the toes. Tapping the feet with the fingertips at the end of the massage energizes the feet.

Massaging the Front of the Body

Lay on your back for this massage. Begin at your feet. The massage will include feet, legs, thighs, abdomen, chest, neck, and face. It will end with the head massage on both sides of your head. Massage for feet, legs, and thighs are similar with a few exceptions.

Temples and Face Massage

Without oil, start moving your fingers or thumbs across the forehead over the temples toward the upper part of your cheeks, a few times. Also move your fingers or thumbs from the middle part of your forehead (in the front) to your temples. Rotate the fingers over the temples a few times

Love   Live   Laugh

before moving them toward the cheeks. Stroke the fingers from the temples toward the cheeks. Repeat these steps a few times. Shake the cheek muscles and temples with your fingers.

Chest and Abdomen Massage

Starting from the shoulders, move the palms toward the chest. Use both palms and move them in sequence one after the other from your shoulders to your chest and from your chest to under your armpits. The massager's palms will move to the middle and the sides of the chest a few times. Move your palms from your abdomen to under the ribcage, but without pressure. Massage sideways a few times. Shake the chest and stomach areas with your fingertips.

Women may also benefit from chest massage. Massage is claimed to help women overcome the symptoms of tumors. The following massages are meant to help reduce tension in the lymphatic nodes under the breasts. Lymphatic stress can be caused by the wires or plastics in a bra. Massage should help release the pressure. The massage involves rapid circular motion of the fingers. Except for the last massage, most can be self-administered.

Chest Massage for Women

The first two steps of this massage can be self-conducted.

1. Using your fingers, massage under the breasts above your ribcage. Start near the middle of your chest moving your fingers outwards to your sides. Make circular motions of the fingers under the breasts and massage almost 30 seconds before moving along to under the other breast. Repeat the movements a few times to relax the area.

2. Massage around the nipples, keeping the fingers almost a half-inch away from the nipple. Move fingers in a circular motion in a

clockwise for 30 second then counter-clockwise direction for 30 seconds, with a total of one minute.

3. This step requires assistance from a massager. As you lay on your side, the massager starts the massage from the side of one breast near your arm. Move rotating fingers upward towards the armpit but along the side. After reaching the armpit, the finger movement changes direction going back toward the starting point. During these motions of one hand, the fingers of the other hand will also move at the same time in a circular motion along the side of your leg. Second hand rotates and moves fingers in a line from the groin toward the knee. Both hands will move simultaneously for 30 seconds on each side of your body. Massage the other side the same way for 30 seconds. (Since this massage step requires both hands simultaneously, it will be helpful to have a massager's assistance.)

Leg and Thigh Massage

Before starting this massage, stretch your legs and notice if your legs or calves are lifted from the surface. If yes, place a pillow or a soft support under the lifted part of the legs. This will remove unnecessary pressure on your back. You may require someone else to massage your thighs.

Massage the thighs, one at a time, with the palms following each other and moving from side to side. The palms keep moving from the top of the thigh toward the knee. Apply no pressure onto the knees. Repeat the massage a few times on each thigh.

Raise one knee, supporting its foot on the massage table or on the ground. Massage the calf from knee to ankle. The massager places her hand under your foot and raises your knee toward your pelvis with light pressure to stretch that region. Repeat this practice twice for each foot. Stretch the legs, knees and thighs and shake the thighs and calf muscles with fingers to relax them.

Oil Mixture

If you are looking for tonic oil instead of ordinary oil, you may consider a mixture. Mix and shake the following oils before each usage.

6 oz.	Peanut Oil
2 oz.	Olive oil
2 oz.	Rose water
1 Tbsp	Lanolin

Massage helps release muscle stress and stimulates its energy.

When muscles get tight, the muscle "knot" may need to be released. The knot is handled by placing a pointed pressure on it for 20-30 seconds to unbundle the muscles. The muscles will lengthen and straighten alignment in the direction of the fascia, relaxing the muscle strain. This is technically called self-myofascial release.

To determine a knot point, move your thumbs with some pressure in the stressed region. Find a point that hurts the most compared to its surroundings. That point could have a knot and may benefit from the self-myofascial release action described here.

Love   Live   Laugh

Sauna or Steam Room Visits

Visits to a sauna or steam room can help the body to relax further. Limit your sauna visits to 10 minutes. You may utilize this period for other exercises or for a short meditation.

Replenish loss of body nutrients after

or

during sauna.

After sauna, take cool shower for a few minutes to close all open pores and wash off the sweat. Thereafter, take normal shower. My Norwegian friend taught me this technique.

One specialist training session in North Carolina told their clients that they should take an iced bathtub bath after their sauna visit. Also an organization named "OUA Bath & Spa" in Las Vegas built an "arctic room." The arctic room produces snowflakes for their clients after their sauna visit.

Closing pores after sauna will help avoid absorption of environmental virus.

Chapter 17

Managing Pollen & Allergies

Early spring and fall are two critical seasons because there is a lot of pollen in the air which causes allergies. These seasons mark the kickoff of sneezing and running noses. Pollen comes from trees, grass and plants. You may end up with congestion, sniffles, itchy and watery eyes, a skin rash or other similar allergy symptoms. Pollen and mold affect our breathing system and can upset our body in numerous ways. Some of us are more prone to allergies than others.

During the allergy season, physicians get busy prescribing all kinds of allergy medication to those who may have developed an allergic reaction from pollen. These allergy medications have to take their course before you are cured. This book provides a means to avoid getting sick from such environmental allergens.

Pollen may also trigger 'asthma symptoms' which will make you feel sick. Inhaling large amounts of pollen occurs when you are near pollen laden bushes and trees. If you are allergic to pollen, I recommend trying to stay away from such bushes and trees.

Pollen and mold have significant allergens especially for those who are sensitive to them. These allergies stress the airways and constrain the breathing system. When an allergen environment exists, common sense demands us to stay away from it, perhaps by staying inside as much as possible. It is also imperative that we clean our nostrils to reduce the pollen accumulation and its effect.

Let's evaluate some of your options to help avoid getting sick from pollen. I have used a Neti-Pot which helped in this endeavor.

Love   Live   Laugh

A Neti-Pot cleans the pollen from the nostrils. The Neti-Pot was introduced to me by my pulmonary physician specialist, Dr. Peter S. Kussin, at Duke University Clinic.

A Neti-Pot reduces the existence of dust mites and pollen that reside inside the nostrils. When pollen gets accumulated in the nostrils, it travels to our lungs with each breath. Cleansing the nostrils is a wonderful way to remove pollen before it can attack your lungs and is essential during the pollen season if you have allergies. Cleansing before going to bed will allow you to breath freely at night and will help reduce the chance of getting sick. Whenever you use a Neti-Pot before bedtime, use it a few minutes before you lay down. This will allow some time to drain extra traces of liquid from the nostrils before you lie down.

A recent medical report stated that if a Neti-pot is used with contaminated water, additional medical problems can occur. If there is a chance that your water may be contaminated, I recommend that you use distilled or boiled water in your Neti-pot. Always use luke-warm water to rinse your nostrils.

The Neti-Pot is available in almost all drug stores and also in Wal-Mart. It is highly recommended that you follow the written instructions on the Neti-Pot. When you are using it, breathe from your mouth and open your mouth slightly during this time. Do not open your mouth wide because this will give you a headache.

The Neti-Pot instructions require that you use the sodium chloride and sodium bicarbonate packages that come with it. You can use either these packages or regular table salt. When using table salt, dissolve ¼ teaspoon of salt in a Neti-pot that is ¾ full with lukewarm water.

I used a Neti-Pot, for the last three years during pollen season. The results have been phenomenal and I did not have an asthma attack.

Love   Live   Laugh

Precaution: Make sure that the water in the pot is just warm and not hot. Hot water will irritate the nostrils.

Hot, dry, and windy weather carry less pollen, however, the pollen count still tends to be higher in the early morning due to environmental moisture. Some things to help reduce sickness from allergies are:

- Healthy food helps make your lungs stronger. Healthy lungs absorb less pollen and dust mites. A link exists between the intake of vegetables and coughing and wheezing. The more you eat, the less it occurs. Eating vegetables and fruits makes a difference. Cherries are considered to be beneficial.
- Omega-3 fats help the lung's cells block inflammation. A good source of omega-3 comes from different fish e.g. salmon, lake trout, albacore tuna, and mackerel. Supplementing your diet with Omega-3 is healthy.
- Stay away from animals and stuffed toys.
- Lower the humidity in your home to help asthmatic conditions.
- Avoid smoking or inhaling secondary smoke.

Throat Irritation

Whenever you feel an inkling of throat irritation and before your throat gets infected follow these four easy steps. These steps will help to reduce your throat irritation. Do them 2-3 times a day.

1. Gargle with warm salted water. Disolve ¼ teaspoon of salt in ¼ cup of tap water. Warm the solution in your microwave oven for 20-25 seconds.

2. Apply Vicks Vapor Rub to the upper chest and your throat. You may also apply it to the outer surface of your nose.
3. Use a Neti-Pot to clean your nostrils as mentioned earlier.
4. Spray Chloraseptic throat spray in your throat.
5. Keep your neck and nose covered with a muffler when the weather is cold.

For an Aruyvedic gargle, mix as below:

One teaspoon - Ginger powder
One teaspoon - Turmeric powder
One teaspoon - Black salt powder
½ teaspoon   - Black pepper
½ teaspoon   - Regular salt

Use a half teaspoon of the above mixture and dissolve it in half a cup of warm water to gargle. Do the step for a few days beyond your recovery.

With self-care, one can avoid pollen related allergies and throat irritation to help you live healthier and lead an active life. Allergies or irritations are not dependent upon your age.

Success Story

In my class, Ms. Pat McElroy, told me, "I used to get a pollen allergy every year. I started using the Neti-Pot in 2005. I have never been sick since. I would recommend the Neti-Pot to anyone any day."

Love   Live   Laugh

Personal Success

My own experience tells me that whenever I feel an itch in my throat or when I sneeze, to use the four steps above. I also drink lukewarm water, coffee or tea throughout the day. My throat irritation has always gotten better.

It was a miracle!!

Neti-Pot and above steps helped.

Chapter 18

Meditation Techniques

Meditation is a very old practice for staying healthy. It is a practice of stilling the mind by controlling the body senses. It relaxes the muscles and reduces both physical and mental stress.

Stress is a reaction to an emotion that may develop from an upsetting caused by jealousy, greed, revenge, lack of sleep, financial problems, actions of others, having a problem with your partner, or due to your poor health. Drugs cannot resolve most of the stress problems. You may seek the help of a psychologist for its resolution. However, why not solve your conflict or problem by using meditation? Meditation will help you to control your mind and may be an easiest path to resolve your mental tensions, by relaxing your senses.

Meditation is a means to release negative thoughts and emotions. By doing so, you help to clear your mind and become physically strong, more alert, emotionally calm and stable. It will change your personality and make you a self-confident, strong, and relaxed person.

Meditation practice improves mental clarity for inner contemplation, concentration, the ability to find creative solutions and understanding the purpose of life. It is recommended that you practice meditation daily for half an hour. Initially it will be very difficult to focus on your thoughts even for a short time. Daily meditation practice will develop achievement of peace of your mind and your capacity to deal with stress, worry, or anxiety. Mental relaxation is the key to staying calm, healthy, happy, and getting your life back on track.

The blood flow, during the meditation, will revitalize your muscles and your brain. The resultant of the meditation will make you feel healthier in both the short and the long runs. With your relaxed mental state, meditation will eliminate your negative moods for a peaceful existence. Meditation becomes more effective you're your positive thoughts (refer chapter: 'Positivity & Happiness').

With positivity, we look for the positive aspects in each occurrence that allows our brain to relax. The combination of stress relief, self-awareness, self-confidence and peace of mind creates a sense within us of well-being. Peaceful thinking brings new revelations and solutions to other problems and will raise your mental level of tolerance to where nothing will unduly bother you. Psychologically mental anxiety relates to emotional problems that develops stress within you.

Since meditation stills the mind by controlling your senses, you will achieve a pleasant mental state with meditation and increase your positive thinking. Such environment will bring the feelings of delight, energy, and ecstasy. To enjoy the fruits of meditation you need to practice meditation daily.

Why daily? Daily practice will help develop your complete concentration. It will help you to reach a state of your mind as is mentioned above. When your body is calm and relaxed during meditation, your breathing will also stay normal and your mind will stop wandering. Meditating on a regular schedule will make you an expert. It will help you to resolve your difficult problem in Stage 3.

Before starting to meditate, you search for a mantra with a pleasant thought of some beautiful element in your life or of your surroundings that you can visualize, concentrate and that will make you feel good. Call this selection as your mantra.

During meditation you will concentrate on your mantra. It will help you to concentrate more effectively and keep your nerves calm during the period of your meditation.

You will recite the mantra again and again during meditation to help you reach your complete concentration. As you mind try to wonder, you will bring back your thoughts to your mantra.

When you are searching for a mantra, you may consider a long string of "OOOOOs" and "MMMs." A long string of "Os" will vibrate your throat as you inhale. A smaller string of "Ms" will also vibrate your throat but differently. At the end of this string you may include words saying "peace & happiness on earth". It will become your mantra. During your recitation you are also wishing "peace and happiness on earth" for everybody.

Your mantra can reflect your "Tolerance, Patience, Existence, Joy, Happiness, Ecstasy, or Peace".

A researcher Megan Rauscher made a presentation at the American Physiological Society in Washington, D.C. Her study explained how Yoga exercises designed by B. K. S. Iyenger have helped reduce activation of the system protein named "NF-kB." Yoga exercises have helped prolong the life of women with breast cancer. Iyengar's yoga concentrated on improving one's posture and reducing the stress (refer Chapter: 'Tips and Precaution'). You need to hold an optimal posture for a considerable length of time to gain and to feel the effects of a deeper penetration of peace.

If you have a physical limitation, you should learn Iyengar's yoga from someone who is trained to teach his methods to the physically handicap persons, instead of attempting to do at your own.

Iyengar's methods point out that yoga posture is an important step. He also helps you to concentrate on your breathing exercises (refer chapter: 'Breathing Techniques') that takes your breathing to a meditative state of mind.

Researchers at Massachusetts General Hospital determined that relaxation techniques such as meditation, Yoga and Breathing exercises turn off individuals' stress genes. The researchers took blood samples from people who habitually meditated for years and examined their gene-expression patterns. More than 2200 genes were activated differently in longtime practitioners of meditation. They also observed differences in cellular metabolism in both longtime and short time meditation practitioners. They concluded that meditation can help in reducing your stress and making your life more interesting.

Buddhists believe that hindrances divert us from the path of getting peace thereby developing restlessness within us.

Overcome mental hindrances such as:

1. Difficulty in concentration → by closing your eyes to help reduce distractions. You may otherwise concentrate on soothing background music.
2. Feeling of anxiety, sadness, or emptiness and lack of self-confidence → by creating and concentrating on some fantasies. Understand them and reduce your frustrations in your life by analyzing with your calm brain.
3. Lack of interest in enjoying or doing things → Change your mental state by changing your work habits and developing a state of enjoyments. Believe in yourself, develop self-esteem and self-confidence. Apply your sincere efforts to accomplish your objectives.
4. Sleeping problems and restlessness → by developing your pleasant mental state and by meditating and concentrating on your breathings in the bed (refer Chapter: 'Sleeping Aids').
5. Feeling tired or irritable → Develop pleasant senses showing patience, flexibility and by developing your energy to deal with all kinds of situations.

Write down any problem that you may think of, that you could not find an immediate solution. In **State 3** during meditation, you may be able to resolve it.

Meditation has **four** States.

Love   Live   Laugh

- **State 1**

  Relax and calm your mind and senses, implies your brain, body muscles, and lymph. To achieve it, you will close your eyes and will concentrate on different parts of your body as is described below.

  Repeat mentally the following words with your feelings. Eventually try to remember them. These steps are based upon Autogenic principles. Allow approximately five minutes for this state.

  a. *"I am at peace and am relaxed and calm"*- repeat 3 times.
  b. *"My arms and legs are heavy"*– repeat 3 times, to relax your arms, and legs muscles.
  c. *"My arms and legs are pleasantly warm"*- repeat 3 times, to help expand the blood vessels for circulation.
  d. *"My heart beat is strong and calm"*- repeat 3 times, to draw attention to your heart beat.
  e. *Concentrate on your breathing* for *one minute*. It brings deep relaxation and helps you to control your breathing to a deeper or a slower breathings.
  f. *"Pleasant warmth is radiating across my abdomen"*- recite the words for *one minute* to radiate warmth across your internal organs, chest and abdomen.
  g. *"My face and forehead are cool"*- recite for *one minute* to feel temperature of your face and forehead in contrast to your other limbs.

  NOTE: If someone is helping you to recite these steps, let him/her read above italic parts while you concentrate on the words and recite them keeping your eyes close. Otherwise, you may open your eyes to read one italic sentence at a time then recite it with eyes close. Continue in this sequence and relax your senses. Try to remember the steps to avoid opening of the eyes.

- **State 2**

    Requires your complete mental concentration while reciting your mantra for *20- 30 minutes* or even for longer periods. Recite mantra continuously with your complete concentration and without any diversion. Whenever your attention get diverted from the mantra, return back to your mantra as soon as possible. Keep on reciting mantra either mentally or vocally to maintain your concentration.

    Your body and brain will unite to clear-of your mental stress. When mind get relaxed, you will think clearly and will solve problems that you may like to resolve.

- **State 3**

    When your brain is calm and rested, as in State 2, you may resolve some complex problem that you otherwise could not solve. Think of various kinds of solutions to help pick the best solution. You will get to this stage only after mastering meditation. This stage occurs, infrequently, after the brain is completely relaxed.

    Calm and clear mind will develop your clear understanding. At the start of meditation, you may skip this state or when you are not seeking to resolve any problem.

    It has been noticed that many of us get new ideas during the night sleep when we are fully at rest.

- **State 4**

    In this state you to return back to your normal-self. Repeat italic steps of **State 1** from bottom up. It means recite them in the order of 'g' to 'a'.

    After completing above steps rub your palms to warm them, and then place them on your eye lids with your eyes still close. Warm your palms once again and then slide them from your eye lids to the sides of your eyes. Open your eyes.

Love   Live   Laugh

Gear your mind towards positive thinking and stops it from wandering to help reduce your stress.

Meditation helps you to conquer loss of your energy, sleepiness, or restlessness.

I was able to help a few with their anxiety attacks, in my classes, by using the meditation techniques.

Posture of Meditation

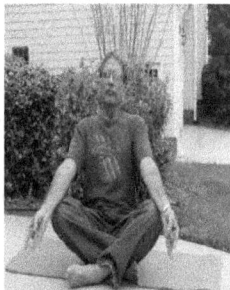

Mostly meditation is carried out in a sitting position on a floor, as shown. However, you may use a chair for your convenience. I believe that a lying posture will put you to sleep. Adopt your optimal posture and feel tall and high in your sitting posture. Keep your spinal cord (back bone) erected with your neck and shoulders stay leveled. You may take help of a mirror for your posture. Posture also requires that your hands rest in your laps with your fingers stretched out as shown.

Ayurvedic science, the oldest and proven science, describes that you press your thumb against the tip of your middle finger during the meditation.

Love   Live   Laugh

Stretch other three fingers outwards in your lap. Ayurvedic method for holding the fingers is practiced all over the world.

Meditation practice does not have to be a solitary activity. You may decide to become part of a meditating group. Benefits of joining such a group:

- Expands your horizon, endurance and self-image.
- Increases your social life and aligns your objectives and emotions with the group.
- Encourages you to continue meditation.
- Encourages you to achieve clarity and wisdom of your mind to help resolve difficult problems.
- Gives you a feeling of security and tolerance.
- Helps develop your compassion for the group.

"We have power within us."

Take advantage of the power that Meditation brings to you.

Meditation brings Tranquility, Serenity, Quietness, Peace, Faith, Love, Joy, and self-confidence.

Love   Live   Laugh

Chapter 19

Sleeping Aids

Physiologically sleep is a natural and essential process of our life, occurring in all humans and animals. It is a complicated state involving both behavioral and physiological processes. Sleep is one of the most important functions that our body uses to regulate, to relax and to keep all our cells healthy. A good night sleep rejuvenates our brain and body cells.

If you imagine or have negative thoughts before going to bed, your subconscious mind will expose to all kind of negativities during your sleep. This will disturb your nightly rest. For a good night sleep, get rid of the negative emotions and think positively.

Before sleeping, turn off all light sources or may use even a sleeping mask. Close your eyes and meditate for a good night sleep. Meditation will revitalize your physical health and in fact, it will revitalize all of your body cells.

Numerous research centers are involved in the evaluation and regulation of sleep with a variety of processes and that includes hormones, neurotransmitters, and peptides. Our brain continues to process information during our sleep as if we are awake. It controls our breathing, heart rate and other body functions.

For individuals who are severely depressed, getting a good night sleep may literally be a lifesaving factor. Body gets much needed rest while your brain stays active. While it is normal to have bad night sleep sometimes, take precautions so that it may not become a chronic problem for you. Usually, poor sleep syndromes need to be dealt at your earliest.

According to a Japanese study, a person who doesn't get enough sleep and has high blood pressure may develop a risk of heart attack, stroke or cardiac arrest. Without an adequate sleep and full relaxation the blood pressure does not dip enough to make you feel rested.

Recent research divided the brain waves during our sleep period into two stages, 'Non-Rapid Eye-Movement' (NREM) and 'Rapid Eye-Movement' (REM) sleeps. As the names imply, the NREM are referred to as the movements behind our closed eyelids with the activities that happen during our sleeping time and REM occurs during when we are in a deep sleep.

Age changes these sleep patterns. Researchers identified these stages by measuring the brain waves. NREM and REM sleep occur for a few times during a one night sleeping period. The 'REM' stage (deep sleep) is absolutely vital for life. The brain consumes increased amounts of oxygen during 'REM' sleep and our heart rates and blood pressure relaxes.

Our projections and neurotransmitters stay active during both periods of 'REM' and 'NREM' and produce a concurrent inhibitory functions and cycle between 'NREM' and 'REM' stages. 'REM' sleep periods occur about every 90 minutes during our sleep period. Our sleep alternates between 'NREM' sleep and 'REM' sleep.

Sleep problems may be due to our physical condition, stress or other factors. When we do not get enough sleep, we will be less alert, less vigorous or more fatigued. These patterns vary with individuals depending upon their neurological development and other related factors. Researchers have shown that lack of sleep may lead to your weight gain over a period and/or may increase your blood pressure. It may also change your thinking capability, your mood and/or your response time.

Love   Live   Laugh

The practice of meditation, as covered in a Chapter: 'Meditation Techniques' that helps individual to sleep without using medication. Meditation requires you to concentrate on a mantra, in this case concentrate on your breathing (inhaling and exhaling). It will facilitate your mental relaxation to help you to go to sleep.

When your brain is disturbed it becomes difficult to sleep or even to concentrate on your breathing. Under these circumstances, take steps to calm your brain activity by concentrating on your positive outlook. Reject any negative thought that may come to you. A combination of positive outlook and concentration on your normal breathing will relax your body and your mood for a good night sleep.

A few suggestions to help you to go to sleep:

- A few minutes before going to bed, entertain yourself with only positive outlooks.
- Relax your brain by staying away from any upsetting subject before going to sleep.
- Schedule and maintain your sleeping time to keep it the same every day.
- Take a warm bath to relax your muscles.
- If hungry, munch some celery and relax yourself. Avoid caffeine loaded drinks before your sleep.
- Whenever you happen to wake up during a night time, return to sleep by concentrating on your breathing. However, if you are trying to remember an idea, write it down on a piece of paper.

The practice of positivity will relax your mind and you will have a restful sleep. Try to visualize that you are in a relax mood, whenever possible.

Love   Live   Laugh

A study pointed out that eating spicy foods, before bedtime, may sometimes disturb you and may result into your poor sleep. In general, avoid spicy foods before bedtime. Spicy foods increase the metabolism and may also increase your brain activity. Intake of caffeine or alcohol can also upset the brain activity for a good sleep.

Keep your bed room temperature at a comfortable level. Desirable room temperature, same sleeping time every day, your positive thinking, and meditation practice will help you with a good night sleep.

There are other factors that can to relax your muscles and nerves. Walk bare-foot, in the morning, on a dew filled wet grass. This natural connection with the earth has shown to relax our muscles.

A CIGNA Wellaware article, in the winter 2009 issue, linked sleep and intimacy. The article wrote, "The relationship between sexual intimacy and sleep goes beyond the fact that both commonly happen in the bedroom. Sex and sleep play a role in your well-being, and each can influence the other. Having sex may help with sleep problems. For some it induces sleep since these are physically and emotionally related. Commit to resolve stress and conflict, including spending time with your partner."

Generally, one needs 7 to 8 hours of uninterrupted sleep daily to maintain your health. Young children, on the other hand, require a minimum of 8-10 hours of sleep. With old-age one may have problems sleeping for longer periods in one shot and thus may spend more time in bed with less actual sleep. It is essential that an older person get total sleep of a minimum of 6 hours in a day to allow healing during the 'REM' phases. Adding afternoon nap to this total and other naps will help to add up the daily requirement of sleep.

The London researcher Francesco Cappuccio writes, "People who get less than 6 hours of sleep each day have 12% more likely chance to die early. Little sleep can develop diabetes, obesity, hypertension and high cholesterol conditions. The relationship between shorter sleep and illness is due to a series of hormonal and metabolic mechanisms."

Again, during a night we go through four to five phases of sleep. As we pass from one phase to the next, we generally do not notice the difference. At the start of your sleep, you may go in and out of sleep – known as light sleep. The thyroids stimulating hormone initially peaks, then continue to decline during our sleep. Deprivation of this activity, due to a chronic sleeping problem, results in an overall reduction of the thyroid function.

After the first phase of light sleep we go to second phase (two) of sleep. In second phase our body begins to rest. The third phase is related to deep sleep in which the body cells will start to recoup to completely relax the body. During fourth phase, our body produces new and additional cells. These cells will break down into proteins. In the fifth phase, our heart rate increases and our brain stimulation start. Finally the blood circulation will rise.

It is recognized that we spend the majority of our sleep period in the second and the third phases. The longer we sleep in these two phases, the more relaxed and fresh we will feel the next day. These two phases are critically essential for our mental and physical health. Tossing and turning during the sleep will make us feel tired the next morning. The fourth phase where additional new cells are generated, will make us feel more energetic.

Once again, the following steps achieve an improved restful sleep:

1. Control your bedroom temperature.
2. Be comfortable and lie with your eyes close. Meditate scanning your relaxed body and muscles and concentrating on your breathing.
3. Stay away from your upsetting thoughts.

Love   Live   Laugh

Direct all your thoughts towards your restful sleep. Above steps will mostly help you to put you to sleep within a few minutes.

Whenever you may wake early, follow the above steps to return to sleep. Help reduce wandering of your mind. If you are unable to go back to sleep, consider that you have enough sleep for that night. Later in a day, you may take a power nap. Avoid going to deep sleep during your power naps. Therefore limit your power-nap time to a half to an hour. Nap period of a half to an hour is sufficient for power-nap that will rejuvenate your energy.

My Personal Aid:

If I happen to wake up in the middle of night, I tell myself that I am still in a deep sleep and my body is completely relaxed. I meditate by concentrating on my breathing as if I am in a deep sleep. This has always helped me to return to a sound deep sleep.

Love   Live   Laugh

Section 3: Unique Exercises to Help Body Pains & Aches

Scope of section 3

The purpose of the exercises contained herein, work to balance and increase your flexibility, stability, and strengthen all of your muscles.

To achieve your fitness objectives, remember to maintain an optimal posture, tall and high, at all the times and breathe through your nostrils. Pull-in your bellybutton with your abdominal muscles while exhaling, during exercise. When we have good health and/or feel physically fit, it is very easy to deviate from correct posture. I can't stress enough, the importance of holding a uniform posture and steady, almost rhythmic breathing while engaging in any exercise. Cardio exercises will also help to strengthen your cardio muscles. This section covers these specifics.

Make a promise to yourself to stay alert and follow these steps to keep yourself healthy, fit and lean for the rest of your life. Increase your motivation by setting a reasonable schedule to engage in exercise. It is critical that your routine covers all different body muscles from your neck down to your feet.

Furthermore, this section presents special exercises not commonly known or practiced. They are extremely effective in targeting pains in the neck, shoulders, back, knees, and legs.

Note the neck exercises include shoulder exercises to help prevent discomfort. For example, many diabetic individuals may suffer from frozen shoulder syndrome. This book provides exercises that will increase the flexibility of your shoulders and of your arms, flexibility of back and other muscles to help you get over the frozen shoulder syndrome.

You may experience back pain relating to the lower part of the spine and associated back muscles. Exercises to recover from such muscular pains are included. These exercises help to reduce lower back discomfort.

Love   Live   Laugh

Lastly, this section addresses leg cramps and spasms. Cramps are mostly related to the muscles in the surrounding region, so by doing the right exercises, you can help yourself relieve sudden cramping.

Did you know that arthritis can start developing at any age? Arthritic pain is the pain of the joints, rather than the pain of muscles. Physicians tend to view arthritis as so common, that they may even seem insensitive to the treatment of such arthritic pains. This section targets multiple exercises to reduce the intensity in the joints, but improving arthritic pain is a long term, that will require your patience. I am confident that with sustained efforts, anyone can improve their situation to a tolerable level.

Finally, the objective of the book is to focus on strengthening your muscles, thereby improving your health and the health of your joints.

Love   Live   Laugh

Chapter 20
Tips & Precautions

Before starting an exercise program, one should be familiar with all the precautions. This book covers a few tips and precautions for your information. (If you are new to the exercise program, start initially with stretches to warm up of your muscles. Take a few deep inhales through your nostrils and exhale through your mouth. Before starting an exercise a few stretches related to the exercise should be conducted. Select repetitions, duration and intensity depending upon your own level of physical ability and goals. Prevent injuries by listening to your body and being sensitive to its needs.

Benefits of Warm-up

- Increases respiratory rate and oxygen exchange capacity.
- Increases blood flow to activate muscles and oxidative capacity of muscles.
- Increases muscle contraction to increase efficiency for contractions and relaxations.
- Increases tissue extensibility and flexibility.
- Increases stability of the muscles.
- Changes heart rate to bring it to your normal level.

Once you have stretched, you are ready to begin the exercises. Stretching will provide flexibility to your body and help you to stabilize, bend, twist, lift and manage bodily movements much more easily. When your body is not flexible, you may end up stressing your muscles when exercising with higher intensity or with too many repetitions.

Love   Live   Laugh

This book does not cover power exercises (anaerobic exercises) that are meant for building muscles for competitions. Rather the book covers aerobic type of exercises that serve to stabilize and strengthen the muscles and joints.

Before selecting an exercise program, first pay attention to your objectives and goals, which should include your plan for health, longevity, and improvement of your self-esteem and physical appearance.

The selected objectives should encourage you to continue with a clear exercise plan. You will need to dedicate time in your schedule for the exercises without procrastination or hesitation. Secondly, select how often you will repeat the exercises depending upon your physique, body condition, objectives and the amount of time you can allocate for the exercises.

Select a program that will achieve your objectives or goals. With your concerted effort, you will observe that in addition to stronger muscles, you will be healthier with the exercises help to rejuvenate your cellular level on up. Motivate yourself to stay with your program and achieve that sensation of healthy and fit feeling. Consider all is fun! Laugh and enjoy yourself.

Your exercise program may also include some aerobics, stretching, yoga and flexing muscles. If you have a personal trainer, will you not allocate time in your schedule for a workout with him or her? You should do exactly the same when you do not have a trainer! Make your routine exercises an important part of your life to optimize your health. Your interest will increase when you include socialization during exercises.

Start with low intensity exercises. Pay lot of attention to your physical condition and listen to your body. Your muscles will get stronger with time due to the changes in the body cells. Pay attention to your inhalations, exhalations, and body posture. As a general guideline when you lift weight or stretch your muscles (concentric contraction) you should exhale and pull-in your bellybutton. When you bring back weight to a starting position (eccentric contraction) inhale and release the stress.

Love   Live   Laugh

Maintaining posture during the exercises is important. You will keep your spine tall and high, keep your feet body width apart and toes in front, legs will be straight, your shoulders will be level and your neck and head will be held up. You may ask why is posture so important?

All neurons and neuron-sensors travel through the cervical spine to our brain for communication between our body and the brain. The sensed information is relayed to the brain which then sends a message back to the muscles to direct proper actions. These muscle actions depend on successful communication along brain-to-muscle pathway. When some obstruction interferes with the sensed information, the muscles may not function properly. To avoid a possibility of obstruction posture is important.

An optimal posture provides us more energy to the ligaments because of proper positioning of ligaments, muscles and spinal bones. Posture helps to alignment, to stabilize and to balance. Out of balance posture will generate pressure on your nerves and may reduce your energy.

Proper breathing and posture are essential for better health. Certain stretches demand proper breathing as part of the exercise. You must master breathing techniques (refer Chapter: 'Breathing Techniques').

I recommend that a workout plan should include different muscle exercises and should spread over a week period. If possible select three to four days in a week for these exercises. Try not to repeat exactly the same exercise every day. To get good results, stretch different body muscles on different days. This will allow you to recoup from the previous day muscle stretches.

Learn to understand your body's needs and limitations. Body will tell you when you are lifting excessive weight or stretching beyond your limits. Follow what your body tells you. That will help you to avoid getting hurt.

Love   Live   Laugh

Coordinate and synchronize your life-style with your exercises without missed days.

- All exercises demand proper breathing. Synchronize your breathing with the stretches and exercises.
a. Inhale to maximum before holding periods is applied in each exercise step. Holding period implies, holding your breath.
b. When you push or lift weight always exhale.

- Repetitions and holding periods and simultaneously remembering may become confusing. You hold to stimulate the muscle fibers. I propose an easy methodology to help this situation.

  Use three sections of each finger to track repetitions and count the holding period mentally. Use first finger to a count of 3. Use the next finger for 4 to 6 count then continue to count on next fingers, as shown here.

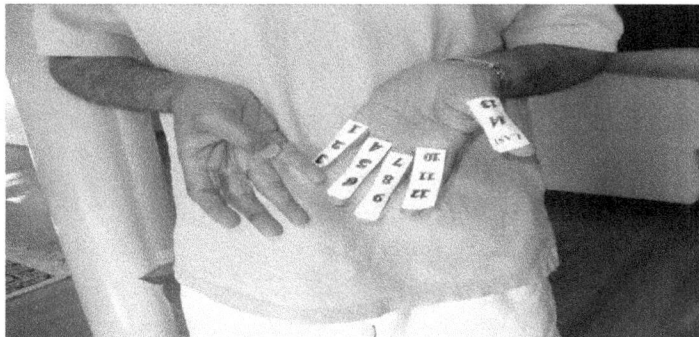

- I usually convert my holding period to an average holding count to represent holding time since it may be difficult to clock during exercise periods.

Love   Live   Laugh

Average count means: counting at fast rate for the period, then counting at a slow rate. Average these counts determine an average count.

- As mentioned earlier, never overstress your muscles, rather stretch them without hurting yourself.
- Learn to balance managed weights when you lift them. Lift weight depending upon your muscle strength.
- Develop the intensity slowly to reach your vigorous goals of anaerobic exercises.
- Allow short rests between aerobic exercises. Whenever breathing gets abnormal, allow longer rest periods till it returns to normal. During resting, inhale slowly over a long period.
- Do not jerk your muscles to lift heavy weights. This action may be harmful than being good. All exercise movements should be smooth and steady. Heavier weights should be lifted for fewer repetitions with longer rests (3-5 min.).
- Keep water or juice handy. When you feel thirsty or dry throat, take a small sip to soothe your throat. Gulping liquids is not recommended.
- Sweating while exercising may cause dehydration or loss of some nutrients. Replenish the loss. If needed, sit calmly under a fan until you return to normal. Thereafter you may finish the remaining exercises, if possible.
- Overcome procrastination by maintaining a regular schedule for your exercises.

Basic advice for an acute musculoskeletal pain

If you feel excessive pain due to some inflammation or overstressing your muscles, you must rest and let the pain subside. Modify your exercise plan and reduce its intensity to help muscles. It may take a few days.

Love   Live   Laugh

Apply an ice compress to the swelled areas for 5 minutes, four times a day and massage the region. You may not stretch the painful muscles for a few days.

When an ice compress alone does not help and if there is no swelling, apply heat compress for 10-15 minutes followed by ice compress. In certain cases, heat therapy may also help.

Heat therapy increases the blood circulation while a cold compress reduces the inflammation. Use your judgment to determine what will help you. Use your physician's advice to select the appropriate therapies.

EXERCISE IS THE ONLY THE REAL FOUNTAIN of YOUTH. IT HELPS BALANCE MUSCLE MASS and BONES.

Flexibility of joints is paramount for connective tissues.

Before starting any exercise program, evaluate your health condition by answering the following questions.

	Questions	Yes	No
1	Has your doctor restricted you from any physical activity?		
2	Do you feel pain in your chest when you perform physical activity?		
3	Did you have had any chest pain in the last month?		
4	Do you get dizzy or lose your balance?		
5	Do you any joint problem that may get worse with physical exercise?		
6	Do you take any medicine for your blood pressure or heart condition?		

Love   Live   Laugh

7	Do you know any reason that you should not do the exercises?		

If answer to any above questions is yes, check with your physician before starting the exercise program. Make sure that it will not hurt you.

Allow time to cool down after the exercises you must. Slow down your exercise before completely stopping.

Benefits of cooling-down: (Minimizes muscle soreness)

- Returns respiratory system to normal
- Avoids dizziness or fainting
- Balances exercises stress

Chapter 21

Neck Exercises

The neck and shoulders muscles are connected by the spinal cord. A combination of cervical and thoracic vertebrae, discs, ligaments and muscles support our shoulders, spine and neck. The tendon of the bicep muscles pass through that area like a rope through a pulley. When you feel pain in either in your neck or in your shoulder, you will essentially need to take care of all of your upper body muscles. Although the book has separate chapters for the neck and shoulder exercises, if you are experiencing neck pain, you can enhance your recovery by doing the shoulder exercises along with the neck exercises. The surrounding to the neck muscles should be flexible. You may pick and choose certain exercises from the list below that helps you the most.

Similar to back pain, neck pain is caused by irritation to the tendons, muscles and ligaments in the upper back and the cervical neck areas. Research shows exercise, massage, and stretching of the related regional muscles will bring flexibility to aid recovery from such discomfort. Stretching your neck using various angular motions and ranges will bring flexibility to your neck and reduce its stiffness.

An abrupt movement of the neck may sometimes cause neck strain. Neck pain due to injury may appear either soon after an accident or after a few days. You may feel it either as neck pain, stiffness, or both. A medical expert or a physician familiar with neck problems should examine your neck before you decide to conduct any neck exercises from this book or any other relief therapy. Knowledge of the neck problem and your neck condition will determine the best route for you to follow.

Love   Live   Laugh

Physicians will generally collect enough data from different types of tests to evaluate your condition. An MRI (magnetic resonance imaging) test is highly recommended since it can pinpoint the exact reason of your neck injury. It may also tell whether it is related to your spine and/or the soft tissue. The MRI is able to visualize the soft tissue such as the cervical discs and upper spine region. There are other tests such as the Electromygram (EMG) or Somatosensory Evoked Potential (SSEP). These tests assist your physician in understanding how your nerves or spinal cord are affected by your condition.

The Somatosensory Evoked Potential (SSEP) test shows the electrical signals of sensation between the body and the brain and is mainly used to diagnose spine problems. The combination of EMG and SSEP tests provides information about how well your nerve roots from the spine column are working. These tests will indicate whether the spinal cord nerves are being pinched or if they are damaged. These tests provide information to determine if you may need a surgical procedure. Before undergoing surgery (unless surgery is the only solution for you) consider conducting a variety of neck exercises which may relax your neck stiffness or help manage the level of neck pain. Avoid unnecessary medicinal or surgical treatments whenever possible, depending upon your tolerance level of pain or discomfort.

Muscular injury or deterioration of the cervical discs causes neck stiffness from time to time. The deterioration of the discs causes a narrowing between the vertebral bodies and may even allow them to rub against each other. Such rubbing will cause a lot of neck pain and may develop a sensation in your arms and fingers. The deterioration of the cervical discs may happen due to aging or misuse of the neck. Whenever you feel numbness or tingling in your arms or fingers and neck pain, it is a condition that will require immediate attention. Consult your spine specialist immediately before any permanent damage occurs.

During the neck exercises, keep your neck vertical and chin leveled to flex your neck. Do not let your shoulders lift or droop during the exercises.

Love   Live   Laugh

Keep your shoulders stationary while you are performing the exercise unless the exercise requires them to move.

Whenever you feel neck pain, practice the exercises below on a daily basis. Your neck pain will return to a manageable level. Setup a daily schedule for your neck exercises. Afterwards, supplemental heat and/or cold therapy may be applied to gain additional relaxation of neck muscles.

Massage improves neck stiffness. Exercises with a rubber band may also help relieve neck pain.

NOTE: During neck exercise, you may sometimes hear a cracking sound in your shoulder joints. Such a sound generally occurs during the stretches due to popping of gas bubbles in the joints. When you hear these cracking sounds and they do not hurt, you may just ignore them. If you get hurt, then consult your physician. In the meantime, rub your neck tendons and neck bones. Follow the exercises properly and carefully.

If for some reason these exercises don't help you, seek the help of a physical therapist, who will determine the affected acupressure points in your neck. Massaging the acupressure points will relieve the neck pressure by releasing the tension in the neck muscles (the process is called self-myofascial release). You yourself can find the acupressure points by applying finger pressure around the neck-pain region and determining the maximum pain point in that region (it is known as the Golgi tendon organ).

To release Golgi tendon tension, apply a lot of pressure with your finger on the acupressure point for 20-30 seconds. Then massage this point. There may be additional acupressure points. Similarly find these points and release their tension.

Ordinarily neck muscle pains will clear within a few weeks of exercising. However, a severe neck pain or cervical disc deterioration may take a much longer time, 1-2 years before attaining a comfort level. Neck discomfort or stiffness may occur often. If cervical discs are deteriorated, the discs will not regenerate, but flexibility will keep neck pain low. Try not to give up easily, no matter how long it may take to get better.

It has been noted that neck pain may sometimes bring on headaches due to neck stiffness. I went through this phase myself. An ordinary headache tablet will cure the headache. It took me almost 15 months before my neck started feeling better. My experience is described in the success story below at the end of this section.

Before starting neck exercises, you will need to acquire a few inexpensive items:

a A stretchable band or string.
b A pair of 1, 2, and 3 lbs. weights.
c A medium or small sized stability ball (balls come in 45-65 cm diameter sizes.)
d A cooling unit and a heating pad for cold- hot therapies.
e Supporting- neck pillows that will provide comfort for sitting on a chair or sofa and also during sleep.

Depending upon your neck condition, the first four items (a-d) are a must while the last item is optional. Some are shown below. During the exercises, you may support your neck with your hands or with a towel surrounding the neck.

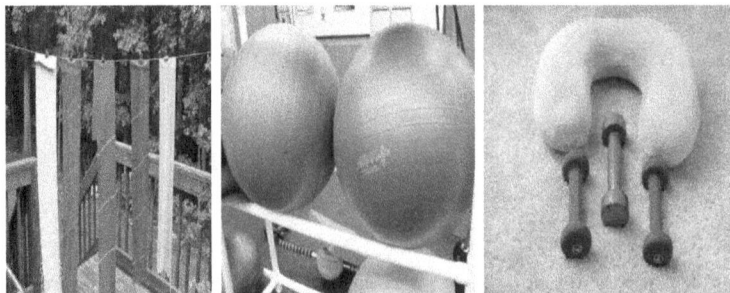

Stretchable bands/Neck Support & dumbbells/Stability Balls

Love   Live   Laugh

Stretchable bands come in yellow, green, blue, red, and gray (low to high tension). Each band has a different density. Select one based on what you can physically handle.

Exercises

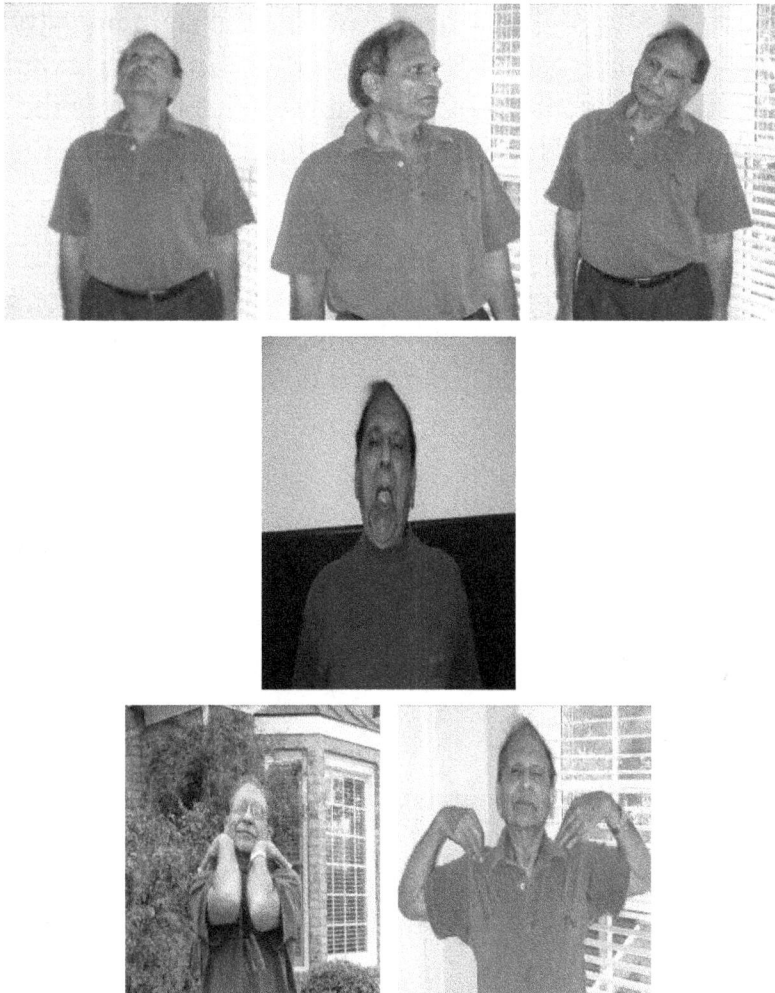

Exercises: To stretch the Jaw – Yawn to open your mouth wide

Love   Live   Laugh

1. Holding your neck vertically, bend the head to look upward. Inhale then hold and stretch your jaw for a count of 5. Exhale and return your neck its normal position. Look downward (your chin is almost touching the top of your chest). Inhale then hold and stretch your jaw for a count of 5 before exhaling and returning. Repeat 5-10 times.

2. Inhale while rotating your head towards the right and stretch the neck over your shoulder. Hold for a count of 5. Similarly exhale and return to your starting position. Inhale again to turn towards the left to stretch over your left shoulder, then hold and count 5. Repeat 10-15 times before returning to the start.

   In the next two steps you will stretch your neck at a 45-degrees angle while looking up or down, inhale and exhale as you move the neck. After stretching your jaw hold for a count of 5, do not bend your head over your shoulder. Keep the shoulders level without rotating them.

3. Turn your neck while inhaling to look up at 45-degrees towards the right. Then hold and stretch your jaw. Turn to look downward inhaling at 45-degrees to your left. Then hold and stretch your jaw for a count of 5. Repeat the step 5-10 times.

4. Similarly repeat the above step, to look up 45 degrees to your left. Then look down at 45-degrees to your right. Repeat the step 5-10 times.

5. Bend your neck over right shoulder inhaling without lifting the left shoulder. Hold there and count to 5 after inhaling. If needed, place your hands behind the back of the neck, without applying any pressure. Maintain your posture. Slowly return your head to the

starting position. Do the same thing on the left side. Repeat 10-15 times.

6. With your chin touching your chest rotate and lift the chin to your right, inhaling. Keep the chin bent close to your chest at all times. Stretch your jaw and count to 5. Exhale and return. Similarly rotate the chin towards your left, inhaling and hold to stretch your jaw for a count of 5. Exhale as the chin returns to the starting point. Repeat these rotations 5-10 times.

7. Place your hands on top of your shoulders. Bring both elbows close to each other in front of you. Rotate both the elbows together, the right elbow moving clockwise and the left elbow moving counter-clockwise. After each rotatation, both elbows meet in front. Rotate both 10 times stretching the shoulder. Let us call this rotation clockwise.

8. Similarly repeat for the counter-clockwise rotation, in which the right elbow will rotate counter-clockwise and the left elbow will rotate clockwise. Rotate the elbows 10 times.

After the completion of the above steps, release the tension of your neck and shoulders by swinging your arms. Swing both arms up and down by your sides, 2-3 times. Twist your obliques at the waist level 2-3 times.

Raise your elbows to waist level and move the arms back and front 10 times. Swing them in a scissor swing; 2-3 times.

Apply hot-cold-hot therapy to relax your neck muscles.

Love   Live   Laugh

During the working day, break your day up by performing neck exercises to relax the neck muscles. Whenever the neck feels pain or stiffness, use the massaging fingers method to massage the muscles and then use cold therapy for 2 minutes followed by warm therapy for approximately 10-15 minutes.

Use of Stretch band or Stretchable string for shoulders and neck

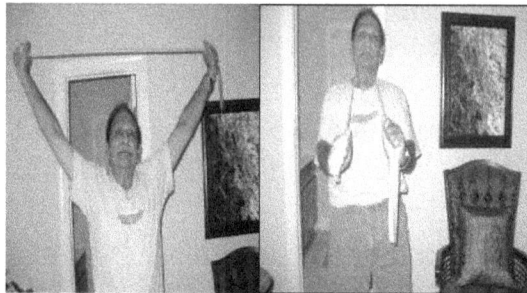

9. Stand tall and high. Hold a stretchable band in both hands above your head forming a V-shape. Stretch the band outward. Hold for a count of 5. Repeat 5-10 times.

10. Hold the band with one hand above your head and hold the other side of the band near your waist. Lower the hand near the waist to go down stretching the band. You should feel the stretch in both the shoulders and neck. Hold for a count of 10. Switch hands to stretch the other side. Repeat 5-10 times.

11. Place something soft to cover the back of your neck. On top place the band holding both its sides. Pull the band down with both hands and

keep your neck straight. Hold pressure on the neck for a count of 10. Repeat 5-10 times.

Neck and shoulder exercises using a stability ball

12. Sit to face the stability ball with your legs under you. Hold a 2-5 lbs. dumbbell in each hand. Rest your chest against the stability ball. Stretch your arms with both thumbs pointing upward. Move your arms down then outward, keeping the thumbs upward. Repeat 10-15 times. You may adjust the dumbbell weights depending on your need. Initially avoid heavy dumbbells.

13. Similarly repeat the above step with the thumbs pointing downward, towards the ground, 10-15 times.

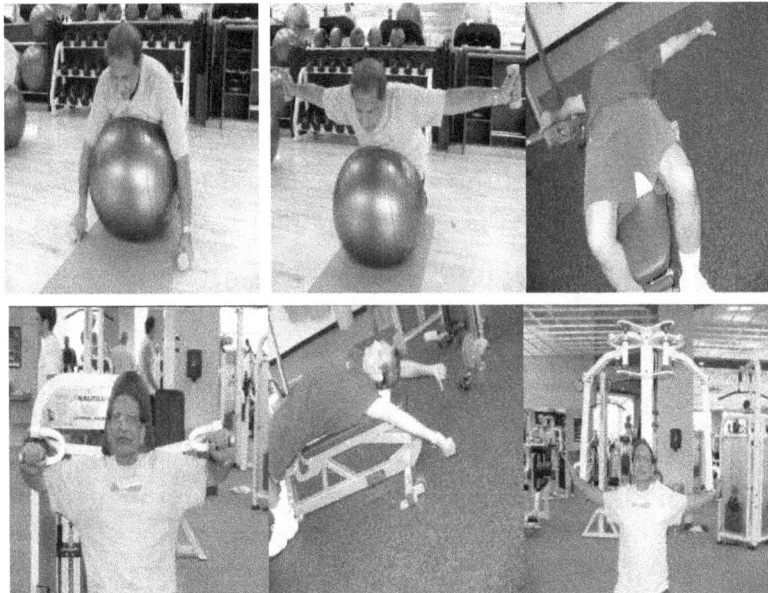

14. In a gym, you may add additional exercises to stretch your back and shoulders.

- o Lie on a workbench and let your neck hang a little at the end of the bench. Stretch your arms out at right angles to you with your thumbs pointing towards your feet. Hold the stretch for 1-3 minutes. Keep the arms as horizontal as possible.

After releasing your arms, cross them above your chest by holding them. Move them up, down, and sideways to release shoulder pressure.

- o Repeat the above step with your thumbs pointing downward and your arms forming a V-shape behind your head. Make the V-shape wider. Hold for 1-3 minutes. After the stretch, cross both arms above your chest and move them up, down, and sideways to release shoulder pressure.

- o Use the Lateral Raise machine, to stretch your shoulders. Set your shoulders in line with the red markings (if any) on the machine. Place the machine pads on your upper arms and lift your elbows to almost in line with your shoulders. Repeat 10-20 times for a set. Relax and repeat 1-2 sets.

- o Use the Deltoid Fly machine to stretch the arms horizontally. Select desired weights and face them. Raise or lower the seat to bring the handles of Deltoid Fly machine at shoulder level. Rotate its bars to your sides as pull your bellybutton inward. This will stretch the posterior shoulders and trapezius muscles. Stretch 10-20 times. Do 1-2 sets.

Love   Live   Laugh

- o Turn yourself 180 degree on the Deltoid Fly machine so that your back is against the weights. Repeat as above for 10-20 to stretch of your Pectoral chest muscles. Conduct 1-2 sets.

You may ask yourself which treatment is better for your neck?

1. Surgery?
2. Physical therapy?
3. Exercises at home with a plan. When needed use small quantity of pain relieving medicine.

You need to make your own decision depending upon your situation.

Personal Success story

This is my neck pain story that will show how I managed my neck stiffness and decreased the neck pain to a tolerable level without having surgery.

I hardly used pain relieving medicine to reduce my pain. The exercises mentioned above and the shoulder exercises helped me. My neck muscles got stronger and more flexible.

Initially, I visited an orthopedic surgeon who diagnosed my neck using a MRI. She concluded that my cervical discs had degenerated due to old age and recommended three options to me.

1. Use prescribed pain killers as long as I have neck pain. She prescribed Ultram 50 mg tablets, one tablet every 6 hours.

Love   Live   Laugh

2. She could send me to a pain killer lab where I would get an injection in my neck four times a year. These injections contain steroids.
3. Have neck surgery. Recovery time - 6 months.

Knowing that the brain nerves go through the cervical area, I decided not to pursue any of these options if I could help it. My belief in the exercises persuaded me to try them first before choosing an option.

I sincerely and carefully followed the neck and shoulder exercises. I also chose not to use medicine unless I had to. Sometimes, I did use one-half or one caplet of extra strength Tylenol.

In addition, I adjusted my pillows to maximize my neck comfort. I used a soft cylindrical neck support which provided additional support to my neck while sleeping. When sitting on a sofa or a chair, I used a neck support to apply pressure to the back of my neck and back. I massaged my neck whenever it became stiff.

Using cold and hot therapies was my savior.

I also used a sauna as heat therapy, for 10 minutes 3-4 times a week. In the sauna room, I exercised my neck. After completing the sauna, I took a cold shower, which I used as my cold therapy and then finally finished showering with a warm shower.

(Note – be careful that in the sauna you may lose some nutrients when sweating. Replenish these lost nutrients.)

My neck pain was reduced by 80% - 90% after 15 months of continuous exercise. My occasional neck stiffness was gone; however I continued massaging my neck. Now my neck feels very comfortable and my neck pain is manageable. I do not need those pain killers any more.

Love   Live   Laugh

Note: Do not give up the exercises even after your neck has recovered from the pain.

I strongly suggest that you evaluate your situation carefully before adopting any program. Seek the help of your physician to determine the cause of your neck pain before you make your own decision for yourself.

Leo a man at my gym had neck pain. I related these exercises to him. He was amazed and he decided to follow them.

Chapter 22
Shoulders & Spine Exercises

Reviewing the upper structure of our body, we find that the cervical cord and thoracic vertebrae (discs, ligaments and muscles) support your shoulders, neck, and spine. They also support each other. Due to such an arrangement of our joints, pain in the shoulders will require attention to the upper top part of your spine and the back. Pharmacists have developed numerous medications to reduce shoulder pain. These medicines are available over the counter or through a prescription from your physician.

Before consuming any medication, consider its side effects. The side effects are not considered good for your body, especially when you consume them over a long period of time. The side effects may be disastrous for you. Some medicines may even harm your internal organs. I suggest that you try to avoid the use of medicine whenever you can. Make your joints and muscles stronger and flexible through appropriate exercise and stretches.

Body exercises, massages, and stretches provide comfort

To your shoulders and joints.

Note: Consider this: after a surgical procedure, your physician sends you to a physical therapist. Your therapist may set a program of exercises for you. These exercises will build and flex your muscles surrounding the affected area. This implies that exercises make muscles strong to bring back their functionality.

Love   Live   Laugh

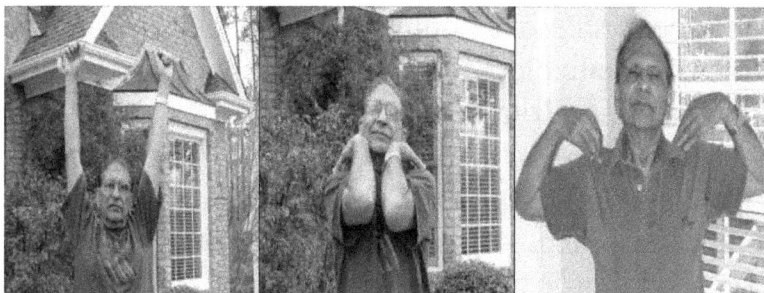

Consult your physician before starting an exercise program.

Shoulder Exercises:

1. To stretch your shoulder muscles, raise your arms above your head. Inhale as you lift your arms and exhale when you bring them down. Depending on your condition, you may be able to hold dumbbells in your hands during the exercise. Stretch 10–15 times. Repeat 2-3 sets a day.

2. Place your hands on your shoulders with the elbows wide open at shoulder level. Exhale as you squeeze the elbows in front of you. Inhale as the elbows return to the starting position. Repeat 10-15 times. Do 2-3 sets a day.

3. Let your elbows come in front of you. Rotate both elbows simultaneously so that the right elbow rotates clockwise and the left elbow rotates counter-clockwise. When these elbows get in line with your shoulders by your side, stretch them backward once then continue to rotate to meet in front. The rotation of the elbows will be a circular movement. Call this rotation a clockwise rotation. Rotate clockwise 10-15 times.

4. Repeat the above step in a counter-clockwise direction in which your left elbow will rotate clockwise and the right elbow rotate in counter-clockwise direction. Rotate 10–15 times.

5. Place your right hand on the shoulder blade. Hold the right elbow with the left hand and lightly pull the elbow towards your head. Exchange arms to repeat a similar stretch on the other side. Repeat each side 5-10 times. Relax a little then repeat as needed.

Exercises with a stretchable band:

These exercises are also covered in the chapter: 'Frozen Shoulders Exercises'.

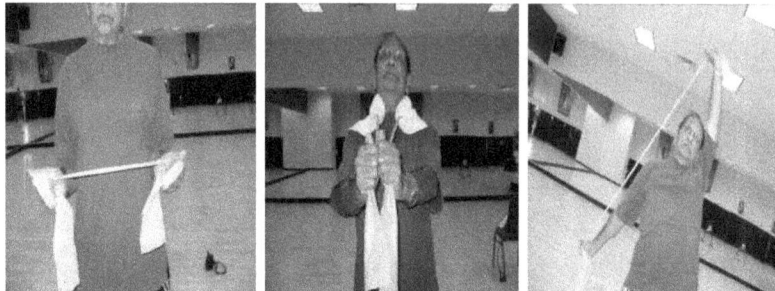

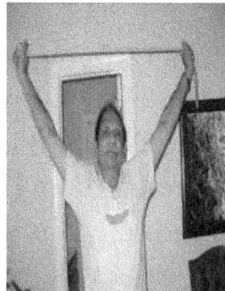

6. Hold the band in front of you so that the width is equal to your body's width. Place your elbows at your obliques so you're your hands are at

90 degree angle to you. Pull the band outward both ways by the twist of your wrists. Hold the stretch for a count of 6, then return.

7. Hold the stretchable band with one hand so that it is above your head and the other hand is near theoblique level. Move the lower hand downward and stretch the band to its maximum. Hold the stretch for a count of 6, then return. Switch hands to stretch the other shoulder. Repeat 15 times each side.

8. Cover your neck with your shirt collar or a towel to avoid rubbing your neck. Hold the band over the collar. Pull the band downward with both hands then release. Repeat 15 times.

9. Hold a band above your head. Stretch your arms upward. Pull the band outward to the maximum forming a V-shape. Hold the stretch then return for a count of 6. Hold a band behind your back. Stretch it outward by twisting your wrists. Hold the stretch for a count of 6, then return. Repeat 15 times.

Upper Spine and Shoulder Exercises

1. Sit on a surface with your feet under you. Bring your elbows to 90 degrees. Lean forward and place the elbows on the surface. Pull your feet back one after the other. You are lying with your stomach on the surface and your shoulders are raised. Your spinal cord is curved. Hold for a count of 30, before lying flat on the surface. Raise your shoulders again and support your spine with the elbows. Repeat 10-15 times.

   Stay lying on the surface and raise the front part of your body by pushing your hands on the surface below chest level. Slide your body forward and backwards slightly, keeping the back arched. Hold each stretch for a count of 5. Repeat 5-10 times.

Love   Live   Laugh

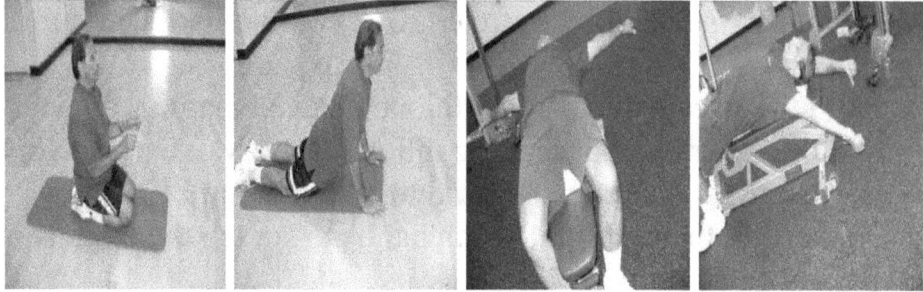

2. Lay with back on a workbench. Lift your spinal cord a little above the bench. Stretch your arms out at 90 degrees and turn your thumbs inward, towards your feet. Hold the stretch for 1-3 minutes.

3. Repeat the above step similarly and stretch your arms behind your head forming a V-shape. Turn your thumbs toward the ground. Increase the stretch as much as possible. Hold it for 1-3 minutes, then return to the starting point.

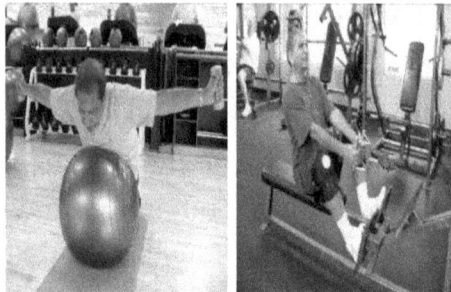

4. Sit on a surface with your legs under your bottom while facing a stability ball. Hold a 2-5 lbs. dumbbell in each hand. Rest your chest on the ball. With your thumbs pointing up, raise your arms outward to shoulder level, then return to the sides of the ball. Repeat 10-15 times.

Love   Live   Laugh

You may choose to use a dumbbell weight depending upon your tolerance level. Initially avoid heavy dumbbells.

5. Similarly repeat the above step with your thumbs pointing downward 10-15 times.

6. In a gym, you may select a multifunctional machine to stretch your upper back and shoulder muscles. Row a tolerable weight at your waist level keeping your optimal posture and exhale to pull-in the bellybutton. You will row by pulling the weight then returning it. Repeat 15-20 times. Relax a little then repeat it again.

7. Sit in the middle of a stability ball with your feet apart. Roll forward until your bottom touches the edge of the ball and your feet are close to the ball. Lay along the curve of the ball with your hands behind your head. Roll the ball backward slowly until your fingers or hands touch the floor behind you. Keep yourself stable on the ball and count 50-100. This will stretch your spine.

To return to the starting position, roll the ball towards your feet slowly until your hands are lifted from the ground. Continue rolling to bring hands above your chest. Next, roll the ball backward to lift yourself to a sitting position.

Stand up to stretch your obliques and inhale. Pull in your bellybutton with each exhale. Repeat the spine stretch on the stability ball again.

Hold a dumbbell in each hand and lift the arms a little by your sides. Rotate the dumbbells clockwise and counter-clockwise 20 times. Rest then repeat.

Love   Live   Laugh

Success story

The above exercises helped Linwood, in my gym. He was suffering from shoulder and arm pain. He had not been able to raise his hands above his elbows. Now he can lift chairs above his head.

Love   Live   Laugh

Chapter 23
Frozen Shoulders Exercises

When the movements of your shoulders and your arms get restricted, it may be a condition known as *frozen shoulder*. With frozen shoulder one feels pain in the upper part of the arms. The pain may get aggravated as the arms move. At times, you may observe inflammation. The ligaments and tissues surrounding the shoulder joints may get stiff due to the acute pain that restricts the arm's movement.

In general, frozen shoulder makes arm movement quite painful. You may not feel like extending or moving your arms. This restriction makes life quite difficult since you may not be able to handle daily chores.

To remedy or correct the situation and to increase the flexibility of your shoulders and arms, exercise the shoulders. Massaging the muscles and stretching your shoulder muscles is a good solution. For massage, refer Chapter 13 'Massaging your Body'. Massage will improve the flexibility of the muscles. Exercise your frozen shoulder by extending and stretching your arms as shown below. The range of of motion eventually increases and it is important to continue with the procedure.

Before starting the exercise, you should massage the stiff muscles with olive oil. Apply hand pressure to your tolerance level during the massage. When you are not able to massage yourself due to restrictive arm movements, you should seek the help of someone else.

How do you avoid a condition of frozen shoulder?

Whenever you feel a slight pain or restriction in your arm movement, begin exercising and stretching your arms and shoulders. Consistent practice

Love   Live   Laugh

of such movements will help your shoulders stay flexible to avoid them from becoming frozen.

A physical therapist told me that his experience and observation tells him, "Diabetic individuals are more prone to the frozen shoulder syndrome." If his statement is true, all diabetics should be more alert and watchful for symptoms of pain or difficulty in the movement of their arms.

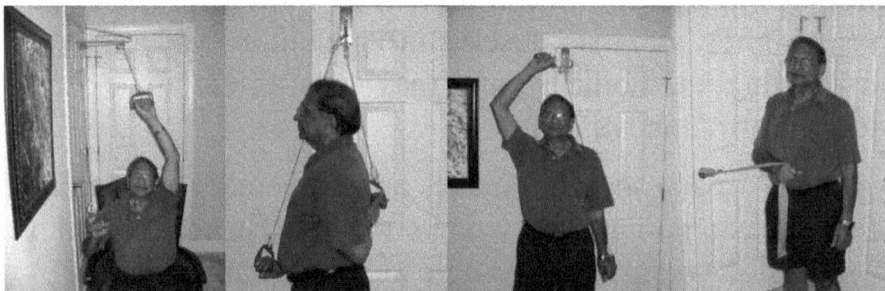

The exercises above and below are quite helpful in almost 95% of the cases. You will need a stretchable rubber band, a set of door pulleys with handles, different dumbbells (1-3 pounds), and a rod about two feet in length. The exercises assume that you own these items or at least these are available to you for your needs.

1. Hang the pulley set from the top of a door. Sit in a chair with both pulley handles in front of you. Adjust the distance between the pulleys and you holding the pulley handles. When you pull down one pulley handle, the other handle goes up, stretching the arm and shoulder muscles. As you pull the left handle down, your right arm will be stretched, stretching the right shoulder. Hold each stretch for a count of 35. Continue alternating arms for these stretches 10 times. Repeat 2-3 times a day.

Love   Live   Laugh

2. Stand with your back to the door near the pulley and put your left arm behind your back holding a pulley handle at the waist level. Hold the other handle in front of you. Slowly but steadily lower your front handle, thereby pulling, raising, and stretching your back arm. Stretch it to a maximum tolerable pressure. Hold the stretch for a count of 35 before releasing. Repeat 10 times. Exchange hands to stretch the other shoulder. Repeat 10 times. Repeat these steps 2-3 a day.

3. Stand with your back to the door. Position yourself holding both pulley handles at shoulder level. Handles are in front of you. Pull the right handle down and the left handle will lift up and stretch the left shoulder muscles. Hold the stretch for a count of 35, then release. Similarly pull left handle down to stretch your right shoulder muscles. Repeat 10 times. Repeat 2-3 times in a day.

4. Anchor the middle part of the rubber band around a vertical pole or a pole of your stairs. Preferably anchor at your shoulder level. Hold both ends of the band without any slack. Face the pole. Pull both ends of the band by raising your hands. Your shoulders will feel the stretch. Hold the stretch for a count of 35 before releasing it. Repeat 10 times. Repeat 2-3 sets a day.

5. Tie one end of the band to a doorknob or to a pole at waist level. Stand sideways to the knob while holding the band in the hand near the knob, without slack. Anchor your elbow on your oblique and pull it away from the knob, stretching the side of your shoulder. Hold the stretch for a count of 35. Repeat 5 times. Turn around 180 degrees, repeat the stretches 5 times. Repeat 2-3 times a day.

Love   Live   Laugh

6. Similar to the above step, hold the band in the hand away from the knob. Anchor your elbow on your oblique. Pull the band away from the knob. Hold the stretch for a count of 35. Repeat 5 times. Turn around 180 degrees, repeat the stretches 5 times. Repeat 2-3 times a day.

7. Stand with your feet body width apart. Curve your right arm over your head, holding one side of a rubber band. Bring your left hand behind your back and hold the band without slack. Raise the right arm up, lifting and stretching the left arm and shoulder. Hold the stretch for a count of 6. Repeat 10 times. Exchange hands to stretch your right shoulder 10 times. Repeat 2 times.

8. Lift your left arm to shoulder level with a band in hand. Bend your right elbow to make a 30 degrees angle to your front. Hold the lower side of the band in your hand without slack. Point your thumbs downward. Then raise the left arm above your head. Hold the stretch for a count of 6. Exchange arms to repeat 6 times. Repeat 10 times for each side. Repeat 2 times.

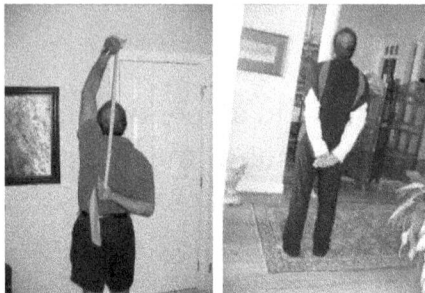

9. Place the back side of your hand on a wall at shoulder level. Slide this hand up with a firm pressure against the wall. Once your arm is lifted,

hold for a count of 10 before bringing the hand down. Repeat with the other hand. Repeat 10 times.

Hold your wrists behind your back. Lift wrists higher and   backward without bending body. Hold the stretch for a count of 35. Repeat 3 times. Repeat 2 sets.

11. Interlock your fingers behind the neck keeping your elbows horizontal to your sides. Stretch the elbows backward. Hold the stretch for a count of 35. Repeat 3 times.

12. Sit in a chair by the side of a table matching your armpit height. Bend your elbow 90 degrees and place it flat near the edge of the table. Apply a firm pressure. Slide your hand forward along the tableside. Go as far as you can go. Hold the stretch for a count of 35. Repeat 10 times.

13. You may stand or lay on a surface holding both sides of a rod in both hands. Hands are spaced equal to your body width. Anchor your elbows against your obliques. Move the rod from one extreme side to the other extreme side 10 times.

14. Lay on your left side. Hold a 1-2 lb dumbbell in your right hand. Anchor the right elbow on your oblique and lift the dumbbell from the floor to your front and twist your wrist upward. Repeat 10 times. Turn to your right side and repeat 10 times. The dumbbell weight depends upon your capacity.

Love   Live   Laugh

Note: It may take you a few months before you achieve your goal after consistent effort. If your condition does not improve, consult your physician.

After the above exercises, apply heat therapy for 10-15 minutes on your shoulders. Heat therapy increases the blood circulation and relaxes the muscles. Massage your shoulders.

Success Story

The above exercises helped my wife's frozen shoulder. It took her 3 months.

Chapter 24
Lower Back

The Mayo Clinic book explains that more than 33 separate bones form the human backbone (spine). A flexible column runs from the base of a human skull to the tailbone. These bones (the vertebras) are stacked on top of one another and in between the vertebras are spongy cushions called discs. Discs have a strong fibrous outer covering that protects the gel inside. A network of ligaments and muscles hold the entire assembly of vertebras and discs. This assembly is called the spinal cord. Back pain may not be due only to a spine problem. There may be other factors, such as an improper curvature at the bottom part of your feet.

An improper curvature of the feet can have a damaging effect on the lower part of your back, knees and legs. It is important that you wear the appropriate type of shoes to create an appropriate curvature in your feet to provide the proper support of your back.

The causes of back pains may be related to the nerves in your back or to the strain on your spinal cord. This book deals only with muscle-related back pains. Muscle pain in the back may also arise without any reason. Other than the exercises and stretches described in this book, your physical therapist should be able to help you to reduce muscle tension. The exercises covered herein are proven exercises that have helped to relieve back muscular pains.

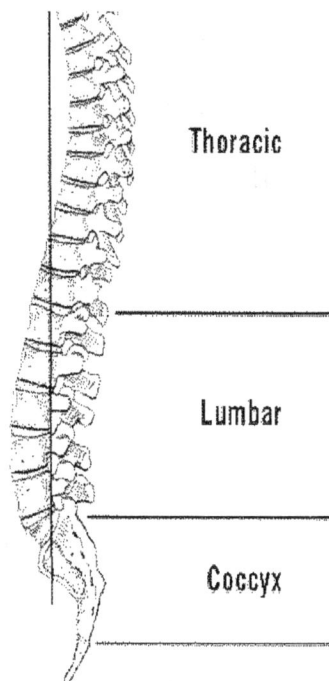

Thoracic

Lumbar

Coccyx

Love   Live

Consult your physician before assuming that the pains in your back are related to a muscular discomfort and to evaluate the exact cause for your condition. If the problem is not muscular discomfort, you may require appropriate medical treatment.

For example, for chronic back problems or disc displacements, you will need specific medical treatment. Most of the time, back pain is related to the back muscles. In men, back pain may also start due to pelvis pain or due to an enlargement of the prostate. Make sure your back pain is not related to any of these medical conditions and is definitely a muscular pain.

Many back muscle pains get better naturally without doing anything. The exercises herein also help almost any lower back pain by strengthening the back muscles. Movements of the joints will nourish and stimulate them by producing the necessary lubrication and allowing the exchange of fluids in the discs. In turn the process builds back muscles, which provides additional support to the spine. One should seek a balanced fitness program which should include specific exercises to strengthen the back muscles. An ideal combination will help regain your body, mind, and back strength.

A common misconception that I hear from many is, "Avoid exercises whenever you feel pain in the spine." Contrarily, the back exercises will help to flex and strengthen the spine muscles.

Strengthen the spine muscles before the back pain worsens. These will also help to avoid your dependence on medication. Remember, all medicine does have some side effects. These side effects may even aggravate other parts of your body. Taking medicine for a short period is generally all right however long term usage or dependence may not be advisable. Strong muscles will support your back and will provide a long term cure for the health of your back.

Mostly back pain strikes when the related muscles are weak or get injured playing sports, an accident occurs, by lifting an extraordinarily heavy weight, or even due to a simple pull of a muscle and a ligament. Examples of muscle or ligament pulls can be a heavy sneeze, getting in and out of your car, sitting in one position for a long period or bending your back incorrectly. Sometimes the back pain may even start with no reason at all. However, back pain should not restrict your activities.

An application of a cold-hot pack to your back may help ease back pain. A cold pack treatment reduces swelling, if any. My experience tells me that a hot pack application for 10-15 minutes, at a tolerable temperature, will do a lot for your back pain. A hot pack lets blood circulate at a faster rate. Hot pack treatments have reduced my recovery time.

When you experience lower back pain or frequent bouts of acute back pain, or a sense that your back pain is going to start, you should slow down your activities a little bit to reduce the strain on your back but you should not abandon them. Resume the back exercises slowly to reduce back stress. You will recover faster when your back problem is at a lower level. Shoulder exercises will also help upper back pain.

When your back is hurting, exercising may not be easy but may become easier by attempting to exercise. Start slowly. Your condition should not discourage you from exercising.

The exercises are good for you. Do not let anything slow you down in their implementation. You may temporarily reduce the repetitions and stress causing elements without completely abandoning them altogether.

It may sometimes take up to 2-3 weeks to feel comfortable. After a short time, your pain will disappear, like magic. Your discomfort period can be reduced with the use of hot therapy. Apply hot therapy, a hot pad for 10-15 minutes, after each session of exercise.

Medicines also reduce back pain without strengthening the back muscles. It's important to build and flex the back muscles often, as they surround the spinal cord to support your body. Back pain can return if the muscles are not strengthened. Among external medicines, you may apply Ben Gay cream or Bio-freeze.

Love   Live   Laugh

Lower back Exercises

The exercises, in this chapter, help all age groups, young, middle and old. These are good for both males and females. Attempt the exercises slowly, carefully, and with some patience. Your dedicated efforts will pay off when your back condition improves. Develop faith in the exercises by reminding yourself that these will improve your condition.

The exercises below will stabilize your lumbo-pelvic-hip complex. The order of these exercises is not as important actually doing them. When experiencing back pain, do these exercises twice a day. After feeling some relief, continue to do them once a day until all pain is gone. At that juncture you may reduce the back exercises to once a week.

Stabilization

1. Lay flat on your back on a surface and stretching your legs and pointing your toes upward. Stretch your toes and legs at the same time and pull-in your navel. The stretche will pull the muscles of your thighs. Hold the stretch for a count of 30-40 and then release. Remain lying for the other exercises.

2. While lying on your back, lift your legs and knees. Move the legs as if you are bicycling. Your toes should be pointing up and your bellybutton pulled-in. Do 20-25 cycles.

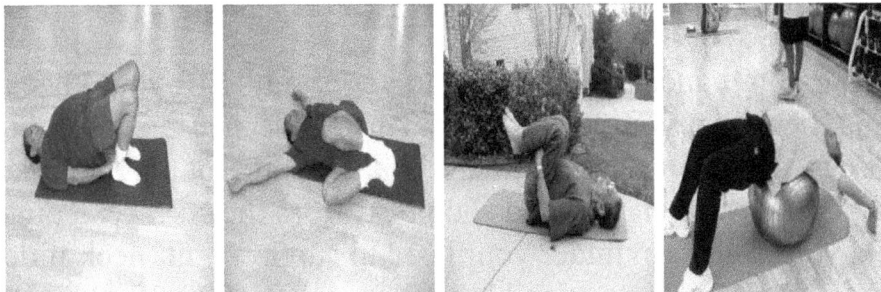

3. Still lying on your back, bring your heels close to your buttocks on the floor. Your feet are parallel to each other. Lift your buttocks upward. Keep your hands facing down by your sides. Look up towards the ceiling. Hold the lift for a count of 30. Return and relax. Repeat 3 times.

Lower back pain muscle exercises and stretches

4. Lie on your back, bringing both heels close to your buttocks. Your knees are together and are lifted. Spread your hands at a right angle to your body with your palms on the surface. Keep looking upward. Bend both knees towards the left and let them almost touch the surface, without lifting your shoulders and hands. Hold the stretch for a count of 20-30 then return your knees to the starting position.

5. Repeat the above step by moving your knees to your right. Again hold the stretch for a count of 20-30 before returning your knees to the starting position.

6. Interlock your fingers under your kneecaps. Pull both knees close to your upper body with your back on the surface. Pull-in your bellybutton. Keep your feet lifted for a count of 20-30. Return your feet to the surface and take a long breath.

7. Spread your hands at 90 degrees to your body. Lift your knees to bring them near your upper body. Turn your knees to the right and as close to the surface as possible. Look up while rotating your knees. Do not lift your left arm and shoulders from the surface. You may hold your right arm under your head to support your neck if desired. Pull-in your bellybutton and hold for a count of 20-30. Return your knees to the starting position but keeping them lifted.

8. Repeat the above step for your other side with your right arm stretched on the surface. Turn your knees towards the left side and close to the surface. Pull-in your bellybutton and hold for a count of 20-30. Return your knees and feet to the surface.

9. Lie with your heels near your buttocks and your knees pointing upward. Place the right foot over the left knee. Clamp both hands under the left kneecap and pull-in your bellybutton. Lift your left knee towards you. Lift your head and shoulder to bring your face closer to your lifted knee. Hold for a count of 20-30. Return your head, shoulders and feet to the starting position.

10. Repeat the above for your right knee and left foot. Hold for a count of 20-30. Return your head, shoulders and feet to the starting position.

11. Sit with both legs under your buttocks. Make a V-shape with your knees in front of you. Your feet in the back will be close to each other. Bend back your upper body so that your head is almost touching the floor. Lay in this position over your legs for a count

of 20-30. This will curve your spinal cord. Return to a sitting position.

Note: If needed, use your elbows to help you go down or get up. Sometimes getting up may not be very easy. In that case, you may roll to your side and release your legs to help.

Repeat steps 4-11 once again.

Relax in a chair with an optimal spinal posture and apply heating therapy to your back for 10-15 minutes.

These exercises will help improve your back pains within 3-15 days as long as long as you do not have any other medical problem and the pain is muscular. For all other reasons, consult your physician.

Exercises with Stability Ball

Select a stability ball with a diameter suitable to you (sizes of 45, 55, and 65 cm diameters). Keeping your balance on the stability ball is essential.

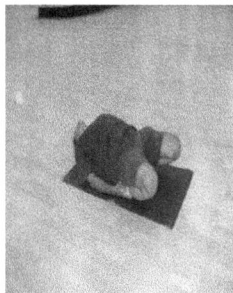

12. Lay on the stability ball with your feet on the surface. Lift a leg horizontally to stretch your back. Hold the lifted leg for a count of

5. Do the same for the other leg. Alternate lifting your legs 15-20 times. Repeat 2 times.

13. Sit in the middle of the stability ball with your feet near the ball. Slowly roll the ball forward until your buttocks touch one side of the ball. Lay on the ball with both hands behind your head. Roll the ball slowly backwards, curving your spine along the curvature of the ball. You may continue rolling back until your fingers touch the surface behind you. Be careful do not to lose your balance. Lay on the ball for a count of 50-100.

   To return follow the instructions carefully. Slowly roll the stability ball forward towards your feet lifting your hands from the surface. Continue rolling forward to bring your arms above your chest. Now roll the ball backward to lift your body to a sitting position. This sequence of actions is important to avoid losing your balance. Repeat 2-3 times.

Personal Success Story

Initially I developed back pain in the 1970s for no reason at all. The above exercises helped me to recover in two weeks. I did not use the heating therapy, but have since learned that heat therapy reduces the recovery period.

I stopped exercising my back after my initial recovery. My back pain returned in 1977 (after 7 years).

I restarted these exercises with heat therapy. My back pain recovered in three days.

In the 1990s my friend, Mrs. Punam Gupta, suffered her back pain. She performing these exercises with heat therapy, she recovered in 3-4 days.

Love   Live   Laugh

Chapter 25

Knee Exercises

Our knees have a complex joint system of muscles and bones. The entire knee joint is held in place by ligaments, muscles, and tendons that are attached to our bones that are located above and below the knees. Our ligament and muscle assembly facilitates the movements of our knees and legs.

According to the Mayo Clinic, if your knee locks rigidly in one position or a traumatic event happens, it will produce intense pain and your knee may cease to function properly. When this scenario occurs you should seek emergency help. A knee injury or the deterioration of cartilage in your knee joint may be a possible cause if you have knee pains. All of these descriptions, however, may not be related to muscle pains. If your pain is due to something other than a muscle related pain, I suggest that you consult your physician.

The exercises in this book relate to muscle pain in the knees. These exercises will build the leg and knee muscles. Stronger leg muscles are known to reduce knee pain. However, you must also check the pronation of your feet because the curvature of feet can also cause pain in the knees. Verify that the knee pain is in your muscles.

A gout condition can also cause knee pain or some swelling in your knees. Your doctor can easily determine gout by checking the uric acid in your body. Gout pains are mostly corrected by adjusting your diet.

Managing the diet reduces uric acid in the body. Ask your doctor for his recommendations for you. The recommendation may include reduction or elimination of certain foods including meat, alcohol, or foods that produce uric acid.

Love   Live   Laugh

Knee pain can also be associated with a restriction in your knee joints. Two bones of the lower part of your leg or the membrane containing lubricants for your knee joints may be inflamed. These two bones are located at the outer base of your knees. In case you feel pain while walking or when bending your knees, it may imply that the knee joints are out of alignment. A misalignment can be related to weak knee muscles. The exercises below will help you strengthen your knees.

Knee Exercises

These exercises can be performed at either your home or at a gym.

Home Exercises

Acquire two weighted belts to wrap around your ankles. When weighted belts are not available, dumbbells can be tied firmly on top of your feet, making sure that the dumbbells will not roll away during the exercises. Choose weights depending upon the strength of your knees.

Use all KIND of PRECAUTIONS

1. Sit in a chair with your back tall and high. Use the belts on your ankles with your toes pointing upward. Lift a leg straight in front of you, stretching it and lifting it close to kneecap height or as high as possible. As a precaution, you should always have a small bend in the kneecaps. Hold the lifted leg for a count of 5, each time. Alternate legs to stretch both knees. Repeat 15–20 times.

   Remove the belts and walk after each round of exercise. Do 2-3 rounds twice a day. Do not stop the exercise until your knee pain subsides. When pain improves, you should be able to lift your toes higher or may be able to hold larger weights. You may also consider reducing the frequency of the exercise, to once or twice a week.

2. Stand near your stairs. Place one foot on the first step and hold the railing of the stairs for support. Bend that knee and move it forward and backward. Transfer your body weight and apply pressure to the knee as you move it. Continue to stretch the knee 15-20 times. Exchange feet to stretch the other knee. Do this exercise twice a day until the knee pain subsides. You may reduce the frequency thereafter.

3. Stand with your legs shoulder width apart and do 10quats. If needed increase repetitions slowly.

Walking on a flat surface or climbing stairs also stretch the knees. As the surrounding muscles get healthier and stronger, the knee pain will go away.

Gym Exercises using the Leg Extension and the Seated Leg Curl machines

Gyms have Leg Extension machines and Leg Curl machines that can be used for your knees. Follow the instructions written on these machines.

The leg extension machine allows you to lift a set of weights. The seated leg curl machine pushes the set of weights downward. You select the weights for your needs.

The leg extension machine builds the upper leg muscles (quadriceps and close to your shins). The seated leg curl machine builds the underside muscles of leg (ham strings).

Love   Live   Laugh

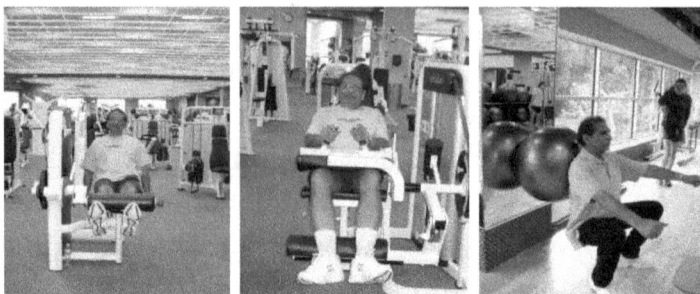

Set selected weights and other machine parameters before placing your feet under the horizontal bar of the machine. The knees should be in line with a *Red Dot* near the edge of your seat on the machine. Lift the weights as high as possible without locking your knees.

Exercises

1. You are a sitting in the machine's seat as mentioned above. If the red spot is not on the machine that you are using, your knees should be at the edge of your seat allowing the knees to bend. Support your back. Lift the bar (lifting the weights) following the instructions for the machine. Hold each lift for a count of 5. Repeat 15-20 times. Repeat 1-2 times per week.
2. After the leg extensions move to the seated leg curl machine. Set the other machine parameters before starting. Follow the machine instructions to position your legs and your back. Place your legs on the horizontal bar. Bring the knees in line with the red spot on the side of the machine. Otherwise place your knees near the edge of your seat. Push the bar all the way down. Repeat 15-20 times. Repeat 1-2 sets.
3. Stand with a stability ball between you and the wall for squats. You may hold a dumbbell in each hand. Roll the ball downward to a squat your (chair-pose). Raise your arms in front of you and keep the spine

Love   Live   Laugh

vertical. Hold the squat for a count of 6 then return to a standing pose. Repeat 10-15 squats. Repeat the set again.

After the pain reduces you may reduce the frequency to once a day for the next 3-4 weeks. Thereafter, you may reduce the frequency to once a week.

Massage your knees after the exercises.

Personal Success Story

Fourteen years ago, I was in Austin, Texas. I started having knee pains.

My physician told me that my knee pain was due to my knee muscles. She introduced me to the above exercises. These exercises cured my knees. When I started the exercises, it was very difficult to lift even 10 pounds. Today, I lift 60 pounds every week.

However, I had stopped exercising my knees after my initial recovery. My knee pains returned. I restarted these exercises. I had second recovery of my knee pains. I do them once a week without fail.

I had helped my friends, family, and neighbors with these exercises.

Additionally I found that walking while holding dumbbells in your hands will also help the knees. I suggest that you add this to the above exercises.

Chapter 26
Leg Cramp Exercises

Cramps in the leg muscles happen suddenly causing a sharp muscle pain. Cramps are usually short and quite painful. We experience leg cramps at different stages of our lives. Often, cramps are an occasional inconvenience and then develop into a nagging problem. At times, cramps may be related to dehydration.

According to the Mayo Clinic, a cramp is actually a muscle spasm in which the tissues contract producing sudden intense pain. A common variety of muscle cramp occurs in the calf muscles during sleep or during prolonged sitting in an uncomfortable position. It may also occur if you stood for a long period at one place. You may get a leg cramp while stretching your leg.

Whenever you are fatigued, stood for long period, wore high heels, or are dehydrated, you may get leg cramp. Lack of potassium in your body can cause a leg cramp. Lastly while stretching your Achilles tendon, you may get Achilles Tendinitis which can cause leg cramps.

Your physician can also evaluate your potassium level during a blood test. If you need to increase the potassium level, drink 6 fl. Oz. of orange juice every day. Orange juice contains a lot more potassium than any other fruit.

The exercises in this book, assume that your potassium level is normal. These exercises, in addition to calf massage, will help reduce the intensity and the frequency of the cramps.

Position yourself so that your body weight is not on your calves before stretching. Stretch your toes away from your calves (moving the toes outward or toeing outward). Toe outward and inward a few times then rotate

Love   Live   Laugh

the toes clockwise and counter-clockwise a few times. The toeing will stretch your calves and ankle muscles. In many instances, the cramp pain will reduce by toeing outward.

However, if starting with outward toeing increases your cramp intensity, start with inward toeing (stretching your toes towards your calves). Inhale and exhale normally during all toeing.

Whenever you have a cramp, start toeing immediately 5-10 times. Then walk and relax for a few seconds before toeing again. After each toeing, walk and massage your calves, your thighs, and inner part of your thighs. Massage helps to reduce the frequency of the cramps.

Whenever simple toeing does not work, lean against a wall while facing it. With your heels on the floor, lift your toes a few times then walk in small-steps. Hold each stretch for a count of 10-30 and repeat 10 times.

Doing toeing exercises even when you do not have cramps helps to avoid them from occurring. Toeing energizes the blood flow in the calves. To avoid cramps during sleep, I suggest that you do toeing and a few leg stretches before going to sleep. Massage your legs often, especially after prolonged sitting at one place to reduce the possibility of a spasm.

Exercises –

1. Stand with your back towards stairs and hold the railing for support. Place one heel on the first stair and stretch your toe up and down. Hold each stretch for a count of 5. Repeat 10 times. Repeat for the other foot.
2. Face the stairs and hold the railing. Place both feet on the first stair. Move the heels up and down by putting pressure on your calves and your ankles. Hold each stretch for a count of 5. Repeat 10 times.
3. Stand facing a wall. Place your hands on the wall. Move your right foot backward and keep it flat on the surface. Lean forward, bending your left knee to stretch your right calf. Hold the stretch for a count of 10. Repeat 5 times. Repeat to stretch your left calf.

Love   Live   Laugh

4. Hold a support. Place your right leg on a chair or on a workbench. Face your leg. Keep your left foot flat on the floor. Slide the left foot backward as far as possible. Stretch your left hands to reach the toes of the right foot. You should feel a stretch in your right calf. Hold the stretch for a count of 15. Repeat 5 times. Repeat for your left calf.

Note: Despite all these exercises and massages, you may still get leg cramps but the frequency and the intensity will be lower.

Make sure that you drink enough liquids to avoid leg cramps due to dehydration. Medical literature recommends eight glasses of water a day.

In females leg cramps may also be related to water accumulation in the feet or swelling of ankles.

Leg pain, especially in the calves and feet, which develops during activity (exercises) and resolves after the activity is stopped is known as intermittent claudication. Intermittent claudication is a distinct form of cramps that occurs only during an activity or the exercises.

The distribution of blood with blood vessels varies considerably with exercise and exposure to heat and cold. It is caused by inadequate blood circulation in your calves and feet and can be arteriosclerosis or P.A.D. (Peripheral Artery Disease). The major arteries, that deliver blood to your legs and feet, become narrowed and blood flow decreases. This can produce cramps in your legs or feet as long as you are exercising. Such problems are common in diabetic persons. Blood circulation conditions associated with P.A.D. is due to coronary heart disease.

Arthrosclerosis describes the condition in which fatty deposits accumulate in and under the lining of the artery walls. Your walk may become lame due to the intermittent claudication cramp.

T.E.D. hose or compression hose socks help leg blood circulation. This hose can be used for short periods. Restrict its use to no more than 2-3 minutes. They can also be worn for a short period before retiring for the night.

T.E.D and compression hose are used to support the venous and lymphatic systems of your leg. They offer graduated compression starting with a maximum compression at your ankles with decreasing compression along your leg. This type of compression of leg muscles aids in blood and lymph fluid circulation throughout the legs. The function of T.E.D. and compression hose is similar.

They are helpful during any type of long trip where you have to sit for a long time with your legs hanging down. You may also practice toeing when you are wearing them. To avoid the legs or feet from swelling you may use them but MUST FOLLOW the PRECAUTIONS.

T.E.D and compression hoses are available with or without a prescription from specialized drug stores that may also sell handicapped equipment. While T.E.D. comes only in white, the compression hoses come in various skin colors.

CAUTION - T.E.D. hose should be used only for short periods at a time. They are meant to help blood circulation in your legs including the calves. For longer usage consult your physician.

IF YOU ARE **DIABETIC** – Definitely consult your PHYSICIAN before using them.

Make sure that you are not suffering from a P.A.D. condition. P.A.D. implies plaque that gets built into the arteries thus narrowing and reducing the blood flow. High blood sugar levels also weaken the arteries and build the plaque. P.A.D. causes leg pains during walks. Old age or family history may contribute to this cause. P.A.D. may coexist with coronary disease or diabetes. Consult your physician whenever needed.

Love   Live   Laugh

Success Story

Carol had calf pain during a bridge session. She told me that she gets cramps every day.

I helped her with these exercises. She was very happy with her success. She decided to help her friends who had similar problems.

I met her after two weeks and she related this success story to me. She added that she had not experienced even a single cramp since I helped her.

Another, Mr. Robert was having leg cramps. He was sitting with pain in his leg. He told me that he fell while playing golf due to a similar leg cramp condition.

I helped him using above exercises. I met him after five weeks. He told me that he was absolutely fine and was very satisfied since he had been playing golf without any problem.

I have seen him many times thereafter but he has never complained about leg cramps or leg pain again.

Chapter 27

Leg or Foot Restlessness

Restless leg syndrome occurs while sleeping. It is a condition in which your legs feel extremely uncomfortable sensations causing you to move your legs keeping you awake. This symptom may last for an hour or so. It is different from getting knee pain or leg cramps. This condition occurs due to Myoclonus contractions that one may confuse with leg cramp.

Myoclonus is twitching of a muscle that usually occurs due to sudden muscle contractions or lapses of contractions. If you experience a jerky motion it may be related to neurological disorders, or it may be an anxiety attack.

Myoclonus gives you the feeling of tingling or pulling sensations deep inside your calves while you are lying down. Myoclonus contractions are not dangerous. You must handle this discomfort or pain to stop its occurrence. Follow relaxation techniques, warm-up therapy and different muscle exercises that will help to stop these contractions. A few steps are:

- Stand with a support, if needed.
- Place a book, nearly 2-3" high and near a wall, place your one toe on the book and heel on the ground.
- Lean towards the wall raising your heel and transferring your weight to the toe. This calf will get stretched.
- Hold the stretch for a count of 15.
- Repeat stretch similarly for your other calf.
- Walk a few steps to release tension in your legs.
- Repeat a few rounds of these steps.

If you are suffering from arthritic stiffness or the musculoskeletal imbalance, you may lose your balance so use a support during the exercise. (The human musculoskeletal system gives the ability to move our muscles and skeleton. It provides a form of body stability to our movements.)

Flexing feet improves the flexibility and the strength for our movements. After each flexing, walk around in all directions - forward, backward and sideways. Maintain your posture during your walks.

For leg and thigh discomfort you can use a different exercise. Lift your thigh parallel to a surface. Hold this position for a count of 5. Switch to your other side and do the same. Repeat for a few times.

You may sit in a chair or stand to stretch your calves. Place your left heel on a bench with your knee stretched out. Place your left elbow on this thigh then bend for your right hand to reach the left toes. Your left side calf will get stretched. Hold for a count of 10. Repeat similarly for your right calf. Repeat 5 rounds for each leg.

Rest in a chair and breathe normally to relax yourself. Massage lower parts of your legs after the exercises.

Chapter 28
Ankle & Toe Spasm

The deep muscles of your musculoskeletal system contract to produce movements at your joints. Muscles are connected to the bones and tendons. When ankle or toe spasms occur, it will immediately increase pain in the muscles that surround your foot.

For instant relief follow the steps below. You may lie in your bed to do these exercises. These are designed to bring fast relief to you from the spasm.

- Allow your foot to move freely.
- Flex your foot inward and outward at a fast rate until the pain subsides.
- After the pain disappears, get up and walk slowly for a few minutes. Lift your heels a few times along the walk.
- Do toeing (refer chapter: 'Leg Cramp Exercises').

When above steps do not bring desired relief to your foot, do the following steps.

- Start in a sitting position where toes are touching a surface and heels are lifted.
- Rotate heels a few times in the left and right anchoring on your toes.
- Now exchange to place heels on the surface and your toes are rotating in both directions.
- These rotations will help. It may take few days to recover.

Foot absorbs all the impact when we walk or run. The Impact occurs as heel touches the ground then transfer all the weight to our foot. Pronation of our foot will disperse this impact stretching our calves. When a foot is flat (without an arch) you will need a support in your shoes to provide the arch and support. Otherwise foot get strained due to insufficient arch that creates some misalignment. Any misalignment of your ligaments, tendons, and muscles should be avoided.

To determine pronation problem in your feet, place your feet on the ground and stand straight. The heel bone (a centerline position), should be upright without the pronation problem. Observe your anklebone when you walk. If your bone leans inward from the centerline, it may be a cause for ankle spasms or pain in your toes.

You may also seek the help of an orthopedic physician. An orthopedic physician should be expert in handling foot tendons. Due to pronation problem, the edge of your heel bone may not take your weight and will cause pains. Foot reflexology is found to be effective for the relief of many ankle sprains and spasms.

Consult an orthopedic physician to evaluate your Achilles, tendons, or pronation needs.

Chapter 29

Bladder Concerns

When the bladder is functioning normally, its walls relax and expand as it fills up with urine. The pelvic muscles and sphincter muscles should stay tight to hold urine in your bladder. When the bladder is full you will decide to go to bathroom to empty the bladder. Afterwards both your pelvic and the sphincter muscles will start to relax.

Again a normal functioning bladder is:

- The bladder wall relaxes and expands as it gets filled up with urine.
- Pelvic and sphincter muscles maintain tightness around the bladder.

The bladder has stretchable muscle walls that may start to weaken with the age or due to the pregnancy or due to some disorder. When muscle walls are weak you may make frequent bathroom visits. In any case, strengthening the bladder and pelvic muscles will help reduce frequent urinations. Ob-gynecologist, Lisa Rankin, MD writes that medication does not work for stress incontinence.

When you develop a bladder function problem that causes a sudden urge or a leak feeling, then your pelvic and sphincter muscles have gotten weak. Due to the stress of incontinence you are suffering from an over-active-bladder situation.

Although this condition is quite prevalent among many elders, age is not a healthy excuse. You should talk to your doctor since the symptoms may be due to some more serious underlying condition, such as diabetes, prostate problems, overweight or some neurological trouble. Your physician can identify these options and can recommend some bladder exercises such as 'Kegel' exercises.

Observe whether your condition is related to the weakness of your bladder muscles, if answer is yes, strengthen your bladder muscles.

Observe –

- If it leaks with bending or standing in a stretch state
- If it leaks during coughing or sneezing
- If it leaks during lifting dumbbells for exercises
- If you are overweight
- If your pregnancy is the cause
- If you are not able to hold when your bladder is full

Your doctor can determine the cause of the leakage.

The bladder exercises below can help strengthening of your pelvic and sphincter muscles and to reduce the bladder urges. Before exercising, determine the correct pelvic floor muscle that needs strengthening. Sense your muscles that need strengthening as follows.

During urination stop in the middle and contract to find muscles that are causing the urges. Quick tightening will determine your pelvic floor muscles. You may use the following steps or you may decide to read "MayoClinic.com" internet site:

- Empty your bladder then lie down on a floor. Keep your knees bent apart.
- Pull in your pelvic floor muscles and hold the pull for three seconds. Make sure that you are not squeezing any other muscle, meaning stomach, legs or buttock muscles. Breathe regularly during the pull.
- Relax all your pelvic muscles for three seconds.

Love   Live   Laugh

- Repeat above steps to pull and to relax 10 times in a sequence.
- Repeat above three times in a day.

Above exercise will help you to get better. Your physician may prescribe some other exercises. Change your lifestyle to meet your needs.

You may go to an internet site to read "MayoClinic.com" site. Where you will go to health information and search for "pelvic Kegel-Exercises".

'Kegel' exercises are known to be the best for fixing your pelvic floor muscles. Drum beat exercise is very similar that can help you to strengthen your pelvic muscles - is described in Chapter: 'Aerobic Stretches'. You may use the drum beat exercise.

In addition, reduce your weight and extra calories. Manage your intake of foods and drinks. Alcohol, caffeinated drink, acidic and spicy foods items cause leaks. Smoking induces cough and become a source of your muscle stress.

This chapter is developed to provide you information regarding bladder concerns. Make your personal decisions after you are medically diagnosis.

Chapter 30

Osteoarthritis Pains

> Every movement puts some pressure on your joints.

Osteoarthritis is one of the most common disorders in which the bone surfaces rub together when the cartilage between the bones has deteriorated. As the bones rub together, inflammation and joint pain set in. This becomes more prominent as you get older. In old age, it is almost inevitable for arthritis to set in. The signs and symptoms are:

- Joint pain
- Discomfort in your joints due to change of weather
- Losing flexibility in the joints and possibly swelling

An arthritic condition implies that the normal flow of body lubricants has decreased and the cushions or cartilage of the joints have deteriorated. The cartilages and discs that provide a cushion in between the joints are breaking down. The bones may have started to rub against each other. Arthritis pain in the spine and cervical vertebrae imply a reduction in the spaces between the bones and this may be the cause of joint or spinal pain. An arthritic condition will bring stiffness and/or swelling of the joints. Consider consulting your medical doctor.

A chronic condition that causes inflammation in the lining of the tissues and the joints is called rheumatoid arthritis. This is also a joint disease that results in joint pain and stiffness. It affects the organs as well as the joints and leads to loss of joint integrity. Managing this disease requires adjusting food habits. Eating a healthier diet may help you. Staying relaxed may also help to prevent the acute flare-ups that occur with rheumatoid arthritis. Rheumatoid arthritis is not covered in this book in detail and I suggest that you consult your physician for additional information.

Living constantly with pain and joint stiffness may interfere with your favorite activities. It does not need to be accepted as a normal part of the aging process. You can take care of these problems, but unfortunately there are not quick fixes or remedies. However, working to make the joints more flexible helps to lubricate them so that they can function normally. Yoga is very useful to accomplish this objective.

This book covers osteoarthritis. Osteoarthritis is related to the degeneration of cartilage of the joints and the wearing of the surfaces of the bones. This condition affects the joints of the hands, knees, hips and spine. Arthritis can inflame and cause pain in your joints. Exercises in this book can help the joint muscles become more flexible and strong. Also use the previous chapters to massage your joints and do yoga stretches. You are trying to achieve:

- Reduction or relief of joint pain for more comfortable living.
- Reduction of joint stiffness.
- Lubrication of the joints and an increase in mobility.

Joint pains are due to variety of reasons. Some joint pains may indicate an arthritic condition, while others merely indicate body fatigue. Arthritis causes wear and tear on your joints leading you to feel uncomfortable. In addition, it may put additional pressure on your joints. Regular stretching of the joints makes them flexible thus resulting in stiffness and pain relief. The range of motion of the joints, as well as the flexibility, will improve. Soaking the joints in warm water will also relax them.

Some medication is available for treating arthritis. Also various natural diets are available to cure arthritis. Natural cures take a much longer period of time than medication. However, natural cures generally do not have side effects which can be a big plus for health improvement and maintenance.

Turmeric and *raisins* are good examples of natural ingredients. You can use *turmeric* regularly with your food; this product is quite prevalent in Japan and India. To use raisins, soak them in rum to swell and consume "*8-10 swelled raisins*" daily over a long period of time. Note: The raisins may take almost a month to swell.

Both of the above dietary suggestions have been successful in reducing joint pain and swelling. I have testimonies from people who have tried them and they will swear by their benefits. Again, if you select either of these methods, you must use them continuously over a few months in order for you to feel an effect on your joints.

Arthritis Exercises:

China developed "Tai Chi exercises" to flex the body joints and to manage arthritis-related pains. Tai Chi exercises stretch the joint muscles carefully, systematically, gently, and very slowly. During Tai Chi exercises, breathe normally. The philosophy of these exercises is similar to yoga, however these exercises are much gentler than yoga.

Tai Chi exercises involve:

- Range-of-motion: Helps maintain your normal joint movements and their flexibility. You learn to stretch your joints and improve the range-of-motion with experience. It is a slow recovery.
- Strengthening: Helps increase muscle strength to support and protect your joints.

Love   Live   Laugh

- Aerobic and anaerobic exercises help with weight control and cardiovascular health. Tai Chi exercises involve only aerobic exercises. If you are lifting weights, weight control is important since excess weight can put extra stress on your joints. Low-impact aerobics (yoga exercises) are recommended for an arthritic condition.

Did you know the most common form of arthritis develops as a result of obesity? Normally healthy cartilage and discs in the body act as shock absorbers for the joints and the vertebrae. Being overweight increases the pressure on the knees, hips and spine. It is essential to manage your weight and to reduce joint stress. Consult your physician or dietician for weight management techniques. Weight reduction will help your joints and in turn will help delay the formation of arthritic pain.

Start gentle exercises to develop your muscles. Most of us fear that stretching the joints will cause additional pain and as a result, discourage you from stretching your joints. This is a misunderstanding.

Change your thinking to allow you to exercise your muscles and aid your recovery. Tai Chi exercises are not intense and are not painful or harmful. However, "Do not expect miracles or immediate results." Continuous effort will eventually be rewarded. Talk to your physician before starting your program.

Movements of Tai Chi exercises, in some ways, are very similar to the movements in martial arts which is well known to us in the United States. These movements open the energy channels in the body. The muscles, joints, and spine benefit from the naturally improved energy flow initiated by the Tai Chi movements. This in turn will help reduce arthritic pain, stiffness, and discomfort. Similar results can be gained by the slow movements of yoga exercises. This chapter combines both types of techniques for your benefit.

Love   Live   Laugh

The wear and tear of the affected joints may occur especially when the protective fluid that cushions the joints is reduced. Regular compression and decompression of the joints may not be very comfortable but these exercises help to improve the absorption of nutrients in the body.

Tai Chi and yoga both require a discipline of breathing and mental concentration. In yoga, the discipline points to the union of breathing, exercise, and mental focus during the exercises. When the three elements are with you, a new world opens up for you. Exercises for your hands, fingers, elbows, arms and feet are described below. For knee exercises refer to the Chapter: 'Knee Exercises'. Immersing yourself in warm water during or after the exercises provides extra relief.

For the Hands and fingers

- Move your hands with your fingers spread in different directions. Twist your wrist and move one hand in front of you. At the same time, move your other hand upward to your side. Twist your wrists in a counter-clockwise motion five times. You will stretch your fingers outward and inward 5 times. After the fingers stretch, close your fists as if squeezing a ball. Switch your hands and repeat. Repeat these movements 2-3 times. You may repeat them as many times in a day as you want to release tension in your hands and finger joints.
- Lift your right arm as high as possible above your shoulders, raising and stretching that hand for a count of 10. At the same time, let your left hand stretch downward by your side. Lift the left hand up near the right hand. Make circular rotations of your hands. Intertwine both hands to lift them higher five times, inhaling and exhaling during this time. Bring your right hand down making circular motions with your hands. Stretch the left arm upward similar to your right hand. Repeat 10-15 times the switching of your arms; inhale with each stretch and exhale during relaxations. Repeat as needed.

Love   Live   Laugh

- Intertwine the fingers of your hands. Stretch your palms outward then inward in front of you. Repeat 10 times. You may also stretch your arms in front of you. You may stretch your arms by both sides and repeat similarly as needed.
- Hold a tennis ball in your hand, and squeeze the ball with your fingers. Stretch your fingers out. Hold the stretch for a count of 10. Relax your fingers by shaking your hands at your wrists. Repeat similarly a few times. If you own a bigger ball you may squeeze the ball with both hands at the same time.

For your Elbows:

Rest your elbow on a cushion at the edge of a table. Hold a dumbbell comfortable for you. If you can't hold a dumbbell, just close your fist without a dumbbell. Stretch only your fist upwards for a count of 10. Hold your elbow along the table. Repeat the same 10-15 times to build your biceps and reduce the elbow pain.

- Hold a dumbbell in your hand. Your arm is by your side, with your elbow resting at your oblique. Rotate your wrist or fist stretching your arm, wrist and elbow in each direction 10-20 times, clockwise then counter-clockwise. This exercise will relieve your elbow pain in a few days.

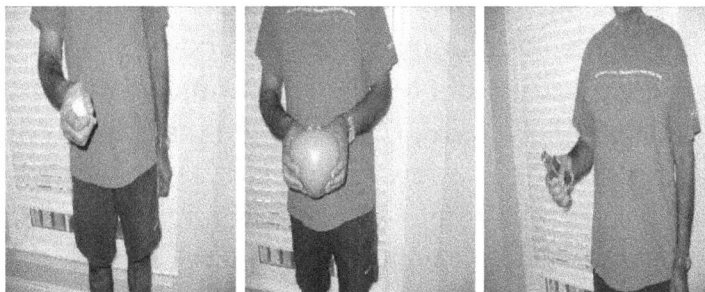

Love   Live   Laugh

- Raise the painful elbow above your shoulders, holding a dumbbell. Let the dumbbell go in the middle of your back raising the elbow high. Raise the dumbbell upward by stretching your arm. Repeat 5 times. Now hold this elbow with your other hand and push it away your head (outward) 5 times. Keep your elbow within your shoulder range. Repeat as needed.

For the wrist

- Hold a small dumbbell and twist your wrist at different angles, meaning you twist your wrist down, to your sides and upward. Repeat 5-10 times.
- Hold your wrist with your other hand in front of you. Rotate your wrist in all different directions. Intertwine your fingers and stretch your fingers, palms and wrists. Repeat 5-10 times.
- Hold dumbbells in each hand. Hold your left hand down by your side and the right hand at a horizontal level in front of you. Rotate both wrists at the same time in all different directions. Exchange your hands and repeat similarly. Repeat 5 times.

Muscle Joint between Thumb and Forefinger

- Massage the hurting part of one hand with your other hand. Apply a coat of olive oil to massage it. Make a round (cylindrical cone) of your other hand with the fingers to cover the hurting thumb and the muscles. Make circular movements in both directions to massage with some pressure. Rotate the cone a few times then stretch this thumb and forefinger backward. Continue the massage of the muscles with your other thumb for a few times.
- Hold and squeeze a round ball and then rest the affected part of your hand. Squeeze the ball with both thumbs a few times. Rest your hand on the ball. Repeat as needed.

Love   Live   Laugh

- You may use a hand squeezer to exercise these muscles. Squeeze often to build muscles and get relief from the arthritic pain.

For the Feet and ankles

- Stand straight, tall and high. Hold the back of a chair to balance your posture, when needed. Place your right foot forward and your left foot in back of you. Rotate your right foot on its toes in all directions. Move the toes of the right foot up, down, and sideways making circular motions wedging on its heel. Repeat similarly a few times. Return to your upright position. Repeat by changing your feet. Repeat as needed.
- Stand as above. Take a small step to your right side. Turn your right foot outward. Raise its heel and squat to touch the toes to a count of 5. Raise your left hand up above your head. Do not lose your balance. Relax a little in your standing position or take a sip of water. Repeat similarly for your left side. Repeat similarly 3-5 times. Repeat as needed daily.
- Sit in a chair and stretch your legs outward in front of you. Move your right foot under the chair and lift your heel on its toes. Bend the right knee to stretch your ankle for a count of 5. Repeat similarly for your left foot. Repeat 10-15 times.
- Stand with some support. Lift your heels. Rotate the heels from side to side in different directions 10-15 times. Repeat as needed.
- Lift your toes up. Rotate the toes from side to side in different directions 10-15 times. Alternate up and down movements. Repeat as needed.
- Use the exercises of the Chapter: 'Ankle & Toe Spasm'.

For Spine

- Stand behind your chair to support yourself. Bend your head back to arch and stretch your spine. Return to your upright position slowly. Repeat similarly a few times.
- Use the spinal exercises of Chapter: 'Shoulder & Spine Exercises' for the upper back.
- Use the exercises of the Chapter: 'Lower Back' exercises for your hips and lower back.

For Legs and knees

- Stand with your optimal posture and use support when needed. Take steps to your front, back, and side. At each step raise your knee to bend at 90 degrees. Hold for a count of 10. Repeat similarly for your other leg. Repeat 20-30 steps in each direction. Repeat as needed.
- In your standing position, lift your thigh to your side, parallel to the ground. Gently slap the lifted thigh with your fist. Lower it. Lay your leg on the chair cushion. Bend to touch your toes with your opposite hand, keeping the knee stretched. This stretches the thigh. Repeat similarly for your other leg and thigh. Repeat 2-3 time. This also stretches the groin muscles.
- Tie both ends of a rubber band around a pole to make a loop. Place your right foot inside the loop. Your left side is toward the pole. With your right foot pull the band away from the pole. This stretches the side of the right leg and the groin. Repeat 10-15 times. Turn around and stretch your left side. Repeat similarly 10-15 times. Repeat as needed.
- With the band still looped around the pole, place your right foot inside the loop. Face the pole. Pull the leg back, away from the pole 10-15 times. Do similarly with the left leg. Repeat as needed.

Love   Live   Laugh

- With the band around the pole, stand with your back to the pole. With your right foot stretch the band away from the pole 10-15 times. Switch to your left leg and repeat similarly. Repeat as needed.
- Sit in a chair and place your right foot on a rubber band. Lift the right foot up by pulling the band towards you. Move the foot towards your right as far as possible. Hold the stretch for a count of 10. Lift this foot above your left knee. Place your elbow on your right thigh and apply a small amount of pressure to lower the thigh. Hold for a count of 5. Similarly repeat for the left side.
- Use the exercises of Chapter: 'Knee Exercises'.

To Relax Muscles

- In a standing posture, inhale and lift up both your right arm and your left leg. Bring your left thigh to horizontal position and your right arm above your head. Lower both of them and exhale. Repeat other side similarly. Repeat 5 times.
- Inhale, rotate and raise both arms in a circular motion by your sides. Let your hands meet above your head. Bring both hands down in front of your chest while exhaling through your mouth. Repeat 5 times.
- Finally, stand in a warrior posture that is stretching your arms at shoulder level, legs and thighs straight with your right foot turned at 90 degrees to your right. Bend to your right side and place your elbow on your thigh. Raise your left arm high. Inhale and hold for a short time. Return to warrior posture and shake your thighs at your sides a few times. Change the warrior posture to your left side and stretch similarly. Repeat 5 times. You may apply a cold pack, if needed.

Yoga and Tai chi stretches help keep arthritis away. Joint massage helps to reduce joint pain.

Love   Live   Laugh

Note: the arthritic pain will return if you stop the exercises. The exercises will keep your joints flexible.

In addition to the above exercises natural dietary remedies are used. As mentioned earlier these are turmeric and golden raisins.

The active ingredient in turmeric is *curcumin*. Our body does not absorb *curcumin* easily but still benefits from it. When you mix black pepper with turmeric, it helps its absorption. While curcumin has anti-inflammatory properties, golden raisins have other pain relieving, anti-arthritic and anti-inflammatory chemicals that may help arthritis and the swelling condition.

Consult your doctor to determine what home remedy will not interfere with your other medicines.

Section 4: Helpful Exercises at a Gym or Fitness Center

Only For your Information

Love   Live   Laugh

Chapter 31
Dumbbell Exercises

Strength training is related to pumping weights, including lifting dumbbells or barbells. Exhale as you lift or push the weight(s) (concentric movement). Inhale as you return to your starting position (eccentric movement). Conduct a variety of dumbbell exercises as described here. Before you begin with dumbbells, make sure that these exercises suit your body and you are not lifting weight that is beyond your limits.

Also, before exercising with dumbbells, stretch a few times and walk on the treadmill for 5 minutes, at your fastest comfortable speed. This will increase your breathing level and make your muscles ready for lifting weights.

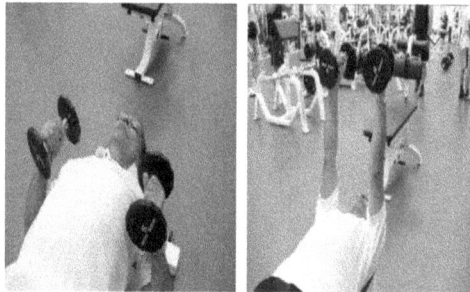

Chest Press and Chest Exercises

1. Lay on a workout bench with dumbbells in your hands. Bring your arms and elbows to your sides, holding the dumbbells parallel to each other. Lift them above your chest. Hold for a count of 10 before returning them to your sides. This works the muscles in the chest. Repeat 10-20 times for a set.

Love   Live   Laugh

2. Continue lying on the workout bench holding dumbbells in your hands. Rotate your wrist as you push them above your chest. (The dumbbells will be in line with each other). Repeat 10-20 times for a set.

Lay across a workout bench with your feet on the floor. Hold one dumbbell behind your head with both hands. Lift and raise the dumbbell above your chest as shown. Repeat 10-20 times.

Forearm and Wrist Exercises

1. Sit on a workout bench as you hold a dumbbell. Rest the arm holding the dumbbell on your thigh. Point the dumbbell down twisting your wrist. Raise it up towards your shoulder for building your bicep muscles. Support your elbow on top of your thigh. Repeat 10-20 times. Switch hands and repeat 10-20 times.

2. Continue sitting on the bench holding a dumbbell. Let your wrist twist downward resting on your knee. Twist your wrist to lift the dumbbell outward and inward. Switch hands to repeat similarly 10-20 times.

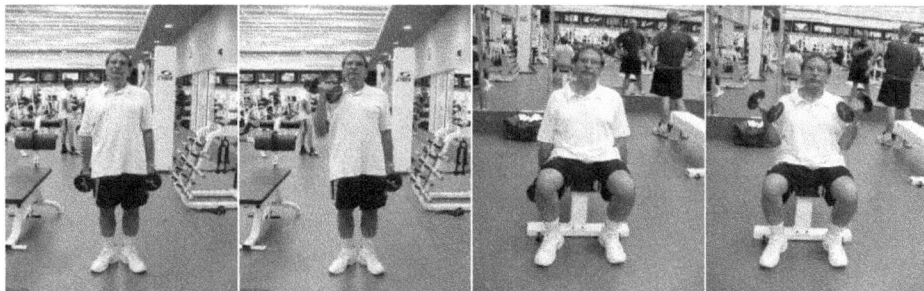

Love   Live   Laugh

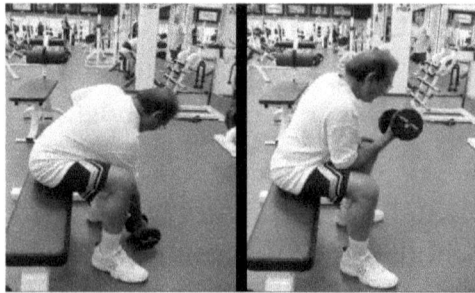

Biceps Exercises

1. Stand in an optimum posture feeling tall and high. Hold dumbbells in both hands. Bend your right arm upward with your hand near your shoulder. Your left arm is down by your side. Bend your left arm up and the right arm down. Repeat 10-20 times for biceps.

2. Sit at out the edge of a workbench, holding dumbbells in each hand and with your hands down by your sides. Lift both hands to your chest level by keeping your elbows touching your waist. Hold there to a count to 10. Repeat 10-20 times.

3. Sit on a workout bench with a dumbbell on the floor in front of you. Wedge your elbow on your thigh and lift the dumbbell to build your biceps. Repeat 10-20 times. Switch hands and repeat similarly for your other arm 10-20 times.

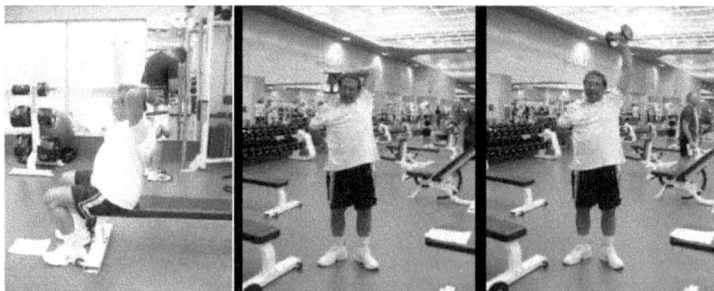

Love   Live   Laugh

Triceps Exercises

1. Sit on the edge of a workout bench. Hold a dumbbell behind your head with both hands. Lift the dumbbell above your head with both hands. Hold to a count of 10 then repeat 10-20 times.

2. Lie across a workout bench, and hold a dumbbell behind your head with both hands. Lift the dumbbell straight up above your chest by stretching your arms. Hold to a count of 10. Repeat 10-20 times.

Stand in your optimal posture, tall and high. Take your right arm above and over your head. Hold a dumbbell. Your elbow is bent over your head. Lift your left arm in front of you at chest level and hold the dumbbell to a count of 10. Bring both arms down. Repeat by switching arms. Repeat 10-20 times.

Chapter 32

Back Workout

Pay attention to your breathing during these exercises. Exhale when you are exerting, and inhale as you release the pressure. Before starting, stretch your back a few times and walk for 5 minutes on a treadmill at your fastest comfortable speed, keeping your spine stretched upright.

Bend one leg on top of a workout bench. Support yourself with your hand on the bench. Raise one dumbbell from the floor to under your armpit. Hold for a count of 5. Return the dumbbell to the floor by stretching your arm downward. Repeat 10-20 times. Switch sides and repeat similarly for your other side.

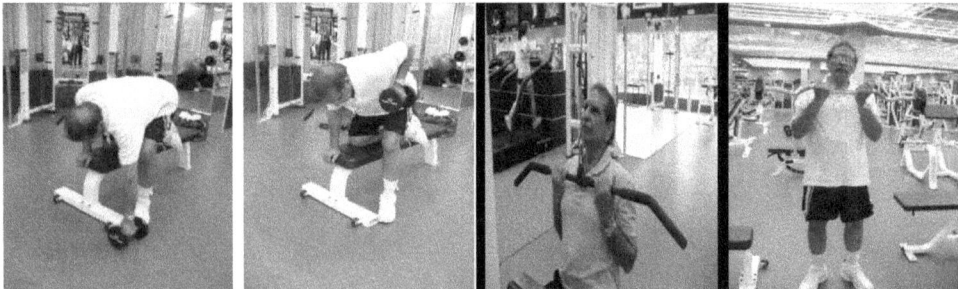

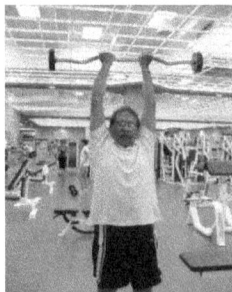

1. Sit erect, feeling tall and high on the workout bench of a multifunctional machine. Select appropriate weights on the machine

for you to pull. Face the machine and pull its bar to your chest level. Keep the bar horizontal. Hold the bar so that your hands are body width apart. Repeat, pulling weights 10-20 times. Similarly repeat when your hands are farther apart on the bar.

2. Load the barbell bar with weights. Raise it to your chest level. Now lift it above your head and stretch your arms. Hold the stretch for a count of 10. Return the bar to chest level. Repeat 10-20 times. This exercise is for your shoulders.

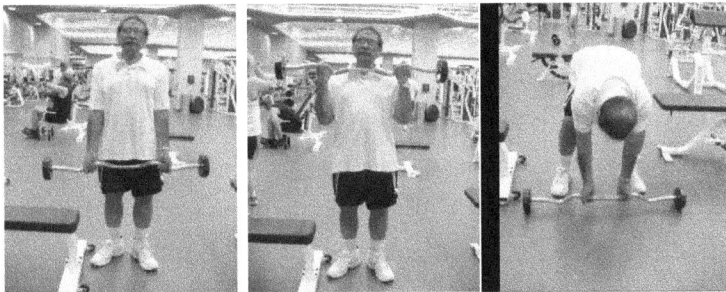

3. Hold weighted barbell at thigh level. Stand tall and high. Lift the bar to your chest level and hold to a count of 5. Repeat 10-15 times.

4. Place a loaded barbell on the floor. Lift the barbell to just below waist level. Your arms are bent in front of you. Hold for a count of 5. Repeat 10-15 times.

5. Stand upright with a loaded barbell in your hands and your arms down. Bend to lift the barbell to your shoulder level with bent elbows. Elbows are kept by your sides. Hold to a count of 5. Repeat 10-15 times.

6. Load a barbell with weights and place it on the back of your shoulders. Be careful not to place the bar on your neck. You may need to bend a little to keep it there. Keep good posture as much as possible. You will feel some pressure on your lower back. Squat 10-15 times.

Chapter 33

Weekly Exercise Program

Exercise is a way to develop strength by strengthening your muscles, flexibility of your muscles and to maintain good health and live a young life forever. Health will bring happiness and stress-free life. You need to exercise muscles of each body part including chest, back, shoulders, calves, ankles and so forth at least once a week, with tolerable repetitions, intensity, and speed. Rest in-between the exercise steps to avoid overstressing your muscles. This program will spread the various exercises over 3-4 days in a week. May conduct 2-3 sets with 10-20 repetitions of each exercise and follow the instructions on the machines. The red parts of the pictures below show muscles that get stretched in each case. Start your exercises as follow:

1. Stretch all parts of your body lightly before starting rigorous exercise. Keep your body flexible and increase your stability. For this you may select, to walk on a treadmill for 5-10 minutes and flex your arms and body in many different directions.
2. Roll your hips on a foam roller for a few times.
3. Practice a few squats.

Above stretches will bring your muscles, tendons, and connective tissues to become active and flexible by pumping upper and lower body muscles, cardiovascular exercises, and all other body muscles to keep you healthy. In addition, control your breathing that will help reduce your stress.

Design your plan to increase the range of your body part movements and to increase their flexibility. Your connective tissues will develop to support your muscles.

Note: the connective tissues take more time to develop compared to the body muscles. Five minutes of treadmill walking at your top comfortable speed will make your tissues active.

DAY ONE (1) Exercises

Start first day's exercises with your shoulder muscles with Lateral Raise. Lateral Raise builds the shoulders and top part of the forearm muscles, as is shown.

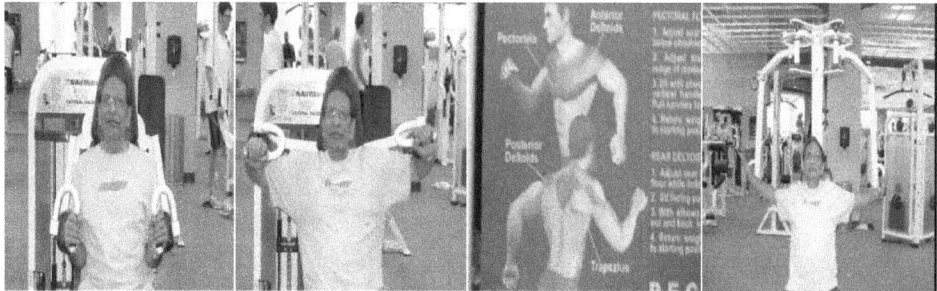

Lateral Raise   Deltoid Fly

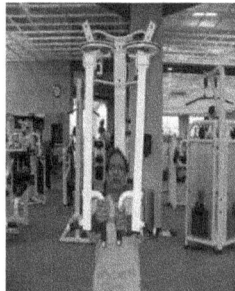

To stretch Deltoid back and Pectoral parts of your chest use Deltoid Fly machine.

Love   Live   Laugh

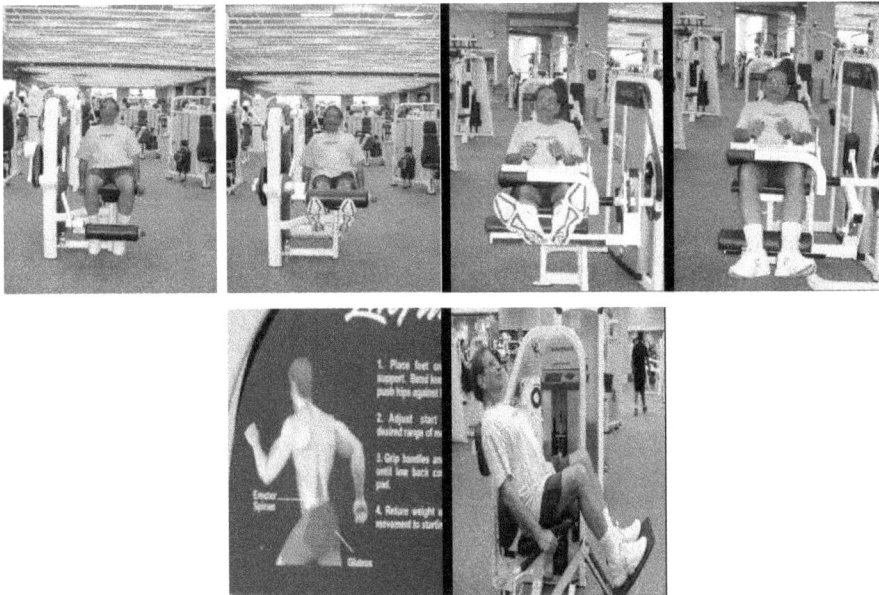

Seated machines for leg are of two types Leg Extension and Seated Leg Curl. To exercise the upper thighs, use Leg Extension machine and under thighs, use Seated Leg Extension & seated Curl machines.

Note: the Erector Spinae, middle lower back does get stretch with Compound Low Row machine. To accomplish it, use Back Extension machine to stretch.

Leg Curl machine, pictures show the top muscles get stretched as you lift the weights and the bottom muscles get stretched as you push the weight down.

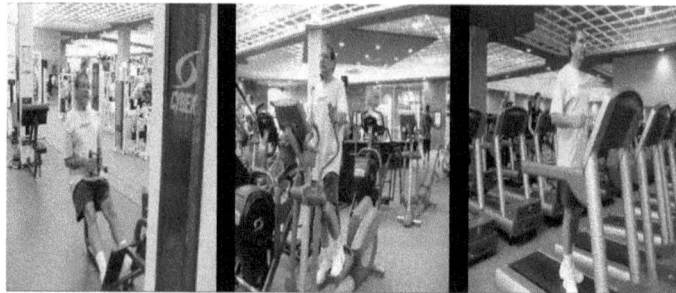

Compound Low Row   Cardio Machines

For Rhomboid and Trapezius back muscles, use Compound Low Row machine to build back muscles.

Cardiovascular exercise are done with elliptical or tread-mill machines. Use each of them at two different times or days during your workouts. Elevate your heart rate on the elliptical 15-25 minutes.

To elevate heart rate on the Treadmill, try to use higher speed walks for 20-30 minutes. Start with slow inclination and slow walks then raising them every 4-5 minutes or more. After allocated time, cool down for at least one minute at slow speed and zero incline.

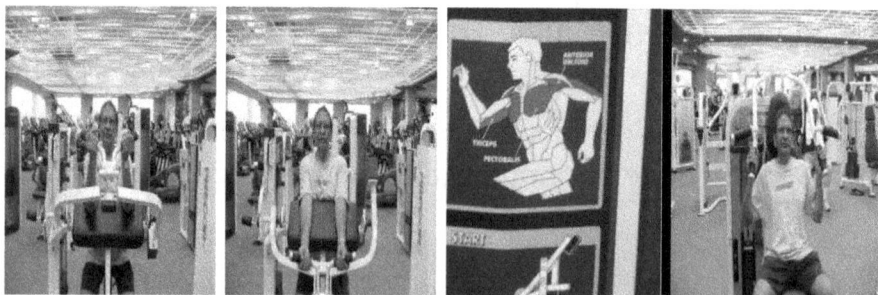

Triceps   Biceps   Iso-Lateral Incline

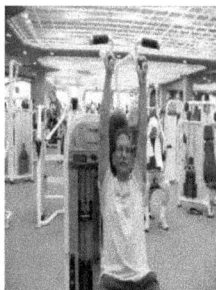

Do other exercises for triceps, bicep, and chest. Use Triceps; Bicep; and Hammer Strength Iso-Lateral Incline Press exercise machines, as shown below.

After completing above machine exercises, you may go to sauna for a maximum of 10 minutes (if facility exists). During this period, you may work out your neck or eye exercises, see Neck and Eye Exercises chapters.

Close all skin pores after sauna visit by a cool shower for a few minutes. You may immediately, thereafter, take a warm shower after cool shower to give your neck a hold-cold-hot therapy.

I learned this from my Norwegian friend. She told me that in Norway, they roll in outside snow after sauna. A specialist training session in U.S., mentioned to their clients that they should take an iced bathtub bath after sauna. Another organization called "OUA Bath & Spa" a center in Las Vegas has an artic-room where their clients go after sauna. In the artic-room, snowflakes were sprinkled. All different approaches have one objective in mind, to help close the body pores that were opened during the sauna.

DAY TWO (2) Exercises

Start as day-one with stretches. On all subsequent days follow similar starts. Your objectives remain unchanged.

Start with ISO-Lateral machine for chest exercises. ISO-Lateral exercises will stretch your shoulders, chest, and biceps.

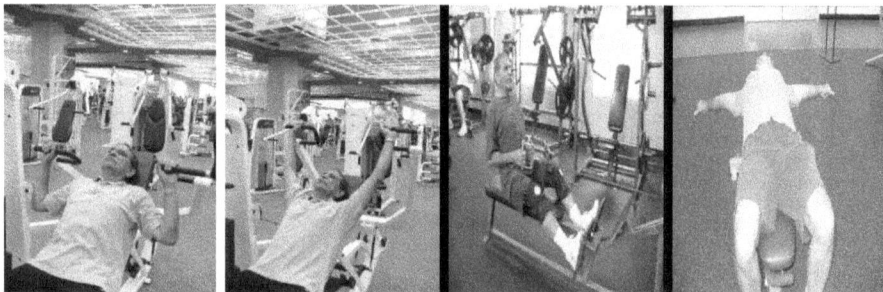

Shoulder Stretches   Back Row   Shoulder Stretches

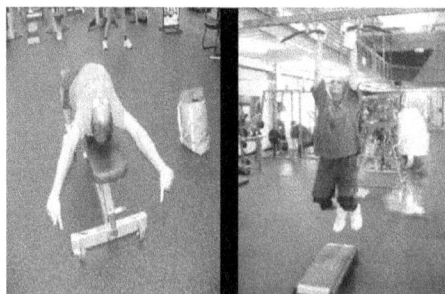

Shoulder & Arm Stretches

Use Multi-functions machine to mix low row exercises as day 1 and shoulder stretches on a bench.

Love   Live   Laugh

Form a V-shape behind head with thumbs pointing downward and enlarge the V-shape to stretch shoulders and feel a good stretch. Hold for 1-3 minutes by counting 100-300. Repeat similar stretch with arms at your sides and thumbs to point inward towards your feet.

Therapists advice to raise the spine by placing some foam cushion under your spine region during above exercises.

Use Multi-functions machine for Low Rowing to exercise the back and the abdomen muscles. Exhale and pull-in bellybutton as you pull the weights. During the pull you exhale and pull-in your bellybutton for abdominal muscles.   Use, as shown, to release strain in your arms by stretching them. You may do it for 15-20 seconds or a count of 50-100.

Exercise legs and thigh muscles with leg-press machine. Use weights that are applicable to you. Hold this weight with each leg individually, by placing foot in the middle, for 15 seconds or count of 50. Thereafter exercise your both legs and thighs by lifting and lowering the weight with both feet placed at hip width apart with toes pointing upward. With Leg Press Machine do 2 sets of 20.

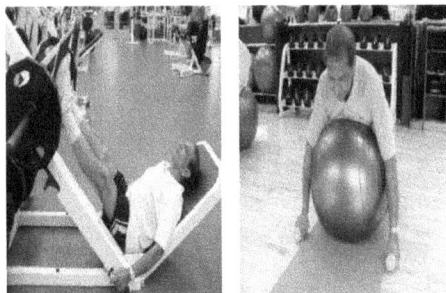

Leg Press   Shoulder Stretch

For a different shoulders stretch, use fig 14. Hold small dumbbell weight in each hand, lay chest on a stability ball. Conduct two sets of 10-15

Love   Live   Laugh

stretches with thumbs pointing downward. Repeat the same stretches with thumbs pointing upward.

Upon completion of above exercises, go for tread-mill cardio and sauna to complete neck or eye exercises, similar to day one. If your gym facility provides steam room, go to steam room and complete breathing and eye exercises. Conclude the exercises with cold and hot neck therapy.

DAY THREE (3) Exercises

As previously, start with Stretches, cardio for the heart and Iso-lateral machine for chest, as day two. Lateral exercises help the back muscles.

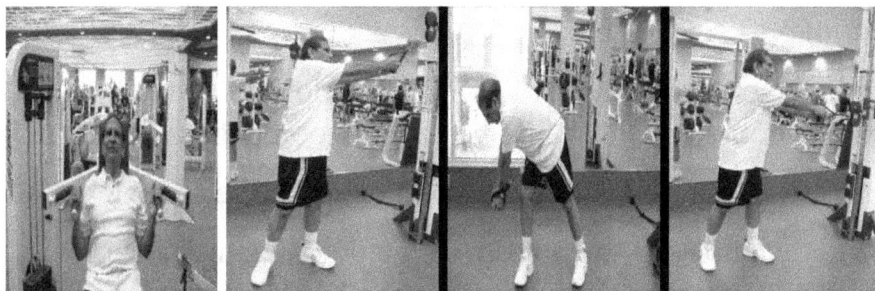

ISO-Lateral Machine   Wood Chops

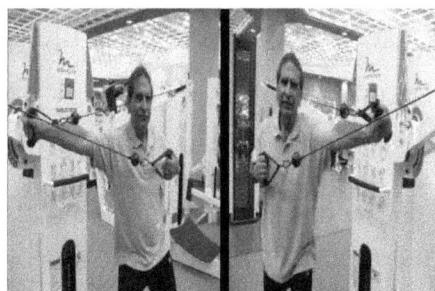

Push – Pull

Next is an oblique exercise and is called the "wood chop" exercise. Use a multi-purpose pulley machine for this exercise. Using both hands, you will pull a rope diagonally, from a position above your head, across your body and down towards your feet. Remember to exhale during the pull, draw your bellybutton inward, and twist your obliques. Set the pulley level at different heights to pull at different heights. Select a desirable and comfortable weight to pull with the rope at each level.

1. Place the pulley at the top of the pole position.

Love   Live   Laugh

2. Stand at the center of the multi-purpose machine with your feet parallel to your body width and facing say north. Pull the weights away from the stack. With your bellybutton pulled inward and your oblique twisted, repeat wood chops 10 times.

3. Turn to face to the south and repeat the wood chop at the same level ten times.

4. Move the pulley to the mid-level of the pole. If needed, adjust the weight for your pull. Facing north, do wood chops ten times.

5. Turn to face south and repeat wood chops at the same level, ten times.

6. Move the pulley to the bottom of the pole. Facing north, do wood chops by lifting your grip to the highest level, away from the weight stack, ten times.

7. Turn to face south. Repeat wood chops at the same level, ten times.

8. Repeat this entire sequence again.

Keep the hands close to each other on the bar for a Lateral pull. Pull the bar to chest level. This exercises the back muscles. During this exercise keep the back upward. Pull 20 times. Repeat similarly by keeping hands at the end of the bar. This will stretch the shoulders and back differently. Repeat both again.

Level-Push-Pull like rowing with both hands and rotating your waistline exercises shoulders, back, oblique, see fig 20. Do 20 times in each direction. Repeat similarly again.

Some abdominal exercises are important for the day. Lay on a stability ball with both hands clamped with or without holding a dumbbell and stretched behind the head. Pull ABS muscles in trying to sit on the ball rotating hands to front. Repeat 40 times twice.

Love   Live   Laugh

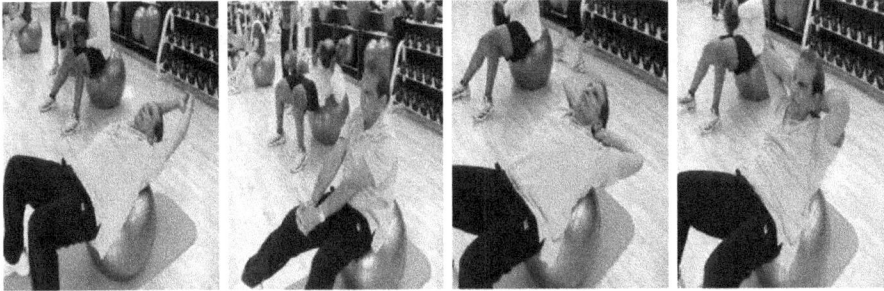

Ab Exercises

After completion of above, go to treadmill for cardio and to Sauna. Do neck and eye exercises and follow the Day-One steps.

DAY FOUR (4) Exercises

Start as previous days then move to abdominal exercises. Balance yourself on stability ball and place hands under neck to support it. Lift shoulders up and pull bellybutton inward by exhaling to stretch the ABS. Repeat 25- 40 times two times.

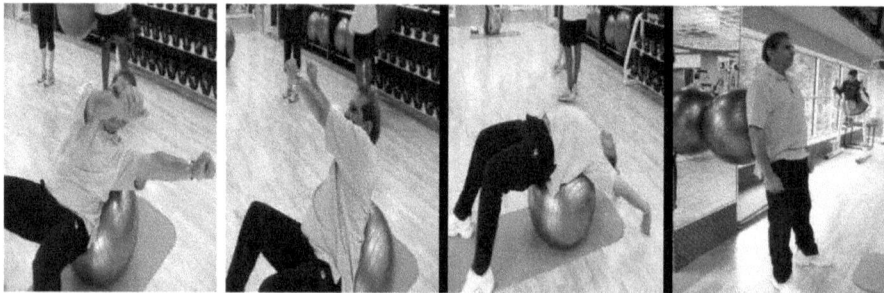

Shoulder Stretches   Spine Stretch Squats Stretch

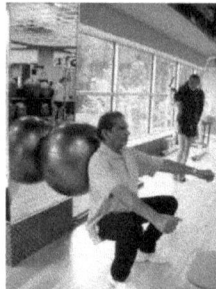

Stay on the stability ball to stretch both sides of your obliques. You may hold medicine ball with both hands to push it away from you. Do 10-15 repetitions in each direction. During stability ball may roll to enhance oblique exercises. Medicine ball helps to stretch obliques.

Love   Live   Laugh

To stretch spine, lie on a stability ball and bring feet near the ball. Roll ball backward to touch hands to surface. Hold to a count of 50-100. To get back is a little tricky. Roll the ball forward till hands lift from surface and are above your chest or your sides. Roll ball backward to a sitting position. Stand and stretch. Repeat it again.

Stand with stability ball between self and wall. Roll the ball downward for squads; pick up dumbbells from surface, and squad with knees bend in a sitting chair pose. Keep body posture tall and high. Hold sitting position to a count of 10 each time. Roll to stand up. Repeat 10 times to exercise knees and thighs.

Other oblique exercises include:

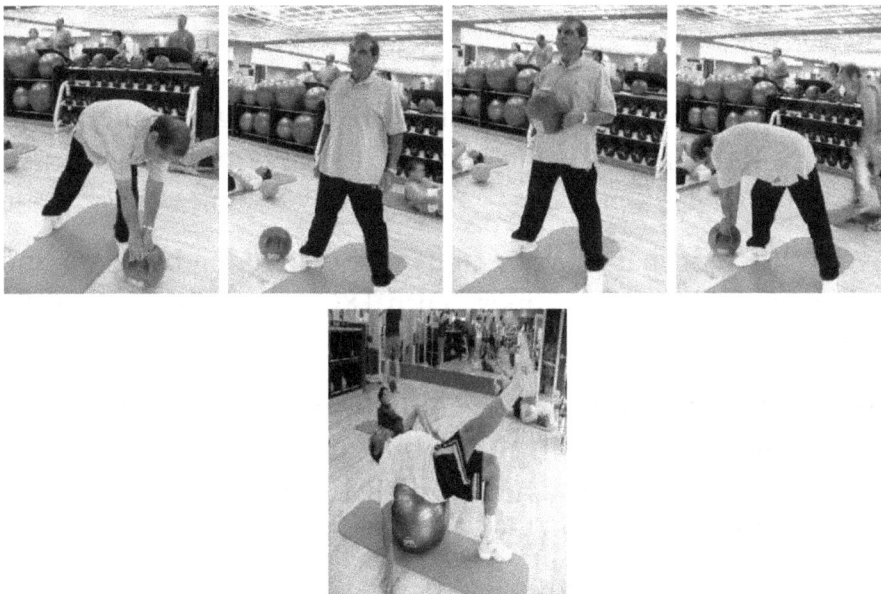

Oblique Stretches

Lift the medicine ball from right surface and standup straight holding ball. Then swing oblique slowly and place it on the left side on surface. Return to upright position without ball. Lift ball from left surface and

Love   Live   Laugh

standup straight holding ball. Then swing oblique slowly and place it on the right side of surface. Return to upright position without ball. Repeat 10 times.

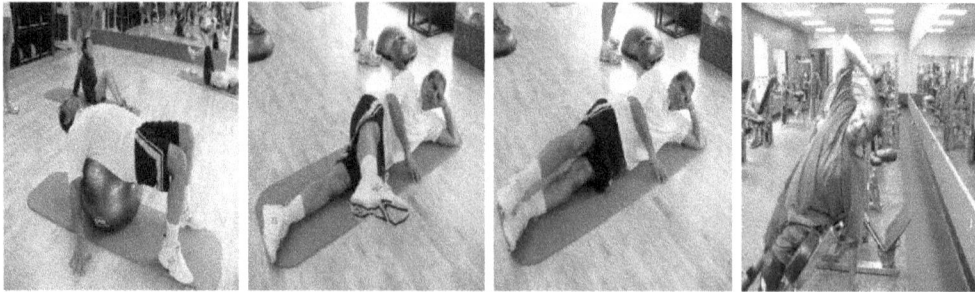

Continue these exercises by lying on the stability ball raising right leg upward. Rotate leg over left leg as far it will go letting oblique roll left. Hold for a count of 5. Return right leg to surface. Lift left leg do the same over right leg. Do 10 times.

Lay on the floor mat by your right side. Move leg back, up and forward to exercise oblique 15 times. Turn 180 degrees and repeat for right leg 15 times.

Lifting arm over-head stretches oblique. On tilt machine lift right hand over head with a dumbbell. Hold 10 lb. dumbbell in left hand. Twist towards left stretching right oblique. Stretch 10-20 times. Turn 180 degrees and stretch left oblique 10-20 times. Stretch both obliques again.

Use Calf Extension to exercise calf muscles and ankles. Adjust weight and seat to rotate feet forward and backward. Push down weights to stretch ankles and calves muscles. Release slowly. Do 15-25 times. Repeat again.

Use Prone Leg Curl to lift appropriate weights towards hips. It will build leg muscles as shown.

Love   Live   Laugh

After completion of above, go to treadmill for cardio, as Day 1 or Day 2. Go to Sauna, steam rooms and showers.

Class Comments

Comments of Jenny Worsley are the following. I thank her for the comments.

"I enjoyed your class and look forward to others. Thank you for sharing your knowledge and experiences. I am pleased to have been asked for my opinion as to what I would seek in a book about Stimuli for Stress-free Healthy Living.

Your suggested title includes the word 'Stimuli' and for me that is the key. I feel we all recognize what we should be doing but struggle to make changes in behavior that will get us there. Can you tell me the answer to that?

I think staying involved with positive thinking and not isolating is a major factor in preventing stress as we age. I will like to read your ideas on this. I enjoyed all your topics during class and see each of those steps to a happy life, no matter what age I am.

Motivation is tough and convincing people to do something for their own good is even tougher. What motivates me is to have a cheerleader/coach that recognizes what I am trying and keeps the encouragement coming.

I look forward to reading your book."

Linda mentioned that her breathing gets heavy during her regular morning walks. Carol said that her stress level accumulates throughout her day. The techniques of this book helped them.

Love   Live   Laugh

References

1. Data and Information from National Institute of Arthritis and Musculosketal and skin diseases- www.niams.nih.gov/index.htm.

2. Information from Arthritis Foundation- www.arthritis.org

3. A new study suggesting drinking plenty of water can reduce the chances of having a gout attack

4. Data and news from National Fibromyalgia Partnership, Inc.- www.fmpartnership.org

5. Mayo Clinic Family Health Book by David E. Larson, M.D.

6. Information from American Dietetic Association

7. Information from American Heart Association

8. Information from National High Blood Pressure Education Program – Information Center/National Cholesterol Education Program Information Center

9. Normal Sleep and Circadian Processes, clinical research paper by Nancy Collop MD, Rachel Salas MD, Michael Delayo and Chalene Gamaldo MD

10. Information from various magazine articles on health, diet, depression and human psychology

11. Live Healthy Article published through EMC Corporation

12. Get Happy and Live Longer article by *U.S. News & World Report*

13. Physical Therapy exercises from many different Physical Therapists over many years of self-experience, including Dunn Physical Therapy for their information relating to many different exercises for neck and shoulders

Love   Live   Laugh

14. Information from American Academy of Orthopaedic Surgeons-www.orthoinfo.aaos.org

15. Well known and published Yoga and Tai Chi exercises

16. Self-experience from my age 10 to now taught by my father, my son, a few physical therapists, chiropractor, and many different doctors

17. Pollen notes are from Fall 2009 literature on living healthy by Medco Health Solutions

18. Quarterly report of CIGNA, Fall 2009

19. University of Florida study regarding nerve cell production in the human brain and how it is directly related to learning and our memory

20. NASM course work, CPR/AED certification, education regarding the function of protein, muscle fibers, and exercise

21. Muscle function as found at www.brainmac.co.uk/musclefun.htm

22. Silver Sneakers Fitness Program provided many stretching exercises for seniors

About the Author

Nature and my surroundings have been very kind to me, helping me to stay fit and learn different ways of keeping myself healthy. I am 75 and have not spent a night in a hospital. Over my life I learned, observed and applied my experiences to maintain my health. I have never been fat or allowed my trim line to get out of shape.

I learned these exercises and their benefits and considered sharing that bounty with you. I believe in helping others to gear their lives towards healthy living. It is up to us to create a happy and healthy environment to enjoy and to benefit from.

I have always kept two objectives in my life: That I will not tell what I do not know, new that I have not tried on myself, and have not analyzed to determine its benefits. When these criteria are not fulfilled, I will respond by saying, "I don't know the answer." I have not really analyzed the needs.

I also believe that if I can help improve the life of even a single soul on this earth I have contributed to do my duty by sharing some goodness with other human beings. I write this book keeping these beliefs in my mind and to reach a larger population who may need my help.

After I retired in 1996 from IBM, I decided to dedicate my life to help others to live their healthy lives. I learned the physiology of humans. I have training equivalent to a personal trainer. I applied my common sense and logical analysis capabilities to evaluate and their relationship between different exercises. I made multiple improvements to perfect them within the realm of this book.

One day I had a dream to accomplish my mission on earth by helping others and to reduce their sufferings, pains, and discomforts. I believe that healthy living is the best solution to live without getting into a vegetative state.

Love   Live   Laugh

My early education was an engineering degrees. My B.Sc. degree is from the University of Delhi. I completed an engineering degree, B.E.E., from IIT (Indian Institute of Technology) in India. My MSEE study was from Purdue University, Indiana.

After the degrees, I worked in the Aerospace Division of Honeywell Inc. in Minneapolis, Minnesota where I analyzed and help the design and the control systems of Gemini, Dynasoar (shuttle of 1963) and Apollo programs, including Swedish interceptor program. All designs and their flight paths depended upon these analyses.

At IBM Corporation, I worked for almost 30 years on various projects. I started as a chip designer and then moved on to a system architect group. I worked as a system designer and a developer of tele-communication systems.

My experience made me an analyst and a logical thinker. I used this background to analyze and to understand, logical, all conditions related to human psychology, physical exercises, and our human physiology. I learned a physical connection with our Healthy Happy Living.

My ideas are presented in this book for you to stay and to live a Healthy Happy Life.

Instructor Spotlight January-May 2011

in the spotlight

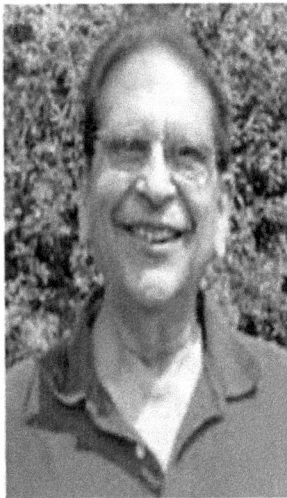

Balraj Aggarwal

Balraj Aggarwal currently teaches seminars on Breathing & Meditation and Happy & Healthy living. His Breathing & Meditation class was even featured on the ABC evening newscast! Balraj also teaches three different levels of Bridge classes, something that he enjoys sharing with everyone! Thanks Balraj!

www.ingramcontent.com/pod-product-compliance
Lightning Source LLC
Chambersburg PA
CBHW081413270326
41931CB00015B/3259